Seeing with the Hands

Seeing with the Hands

Blindness, Vision, and Touch after Descartes

Mark Paterson

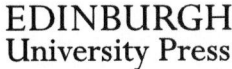
EDINBURGH
University Press

Edinburgh University Press is one of the leading university presses in the UK. We publish academic books and journals in our selected subject areas across the humanities and social sciences, combining cutting-edge scholarship with high editorial and production values to produce academic works of lasting importance. For more information visit our website: www.edinburghuniversitypress.com

© Mark Paterson, 2016

Edinburgh University Press Ltd
The Tun – Holyrood Road,
12(2f) Jackson's Entry,
Edinburgh EH8 8PJ

Typeset in 11/13 Adobe Sabon by
IDSUK (DataConnection) Ltd, and
printed and bound in Great Britain by
CPI Group (UK) Ltd, Croydon CR0 4YY

A CIP record for this book is available from the British Library

ISBN 978 1 4744 0531 7 (hardback)
ISBN 978 1 4744 0533 1 (webready PDF)
ISBN 978 1 4744 0532 4 (paperback)
ISBN 978 1 4744 0534 8 (epub)

The right of Mark Paterson to be identified as the author of this work has been asserted in accordance with the Copyright, Designs and Patents Act 1988, and the Copyright and Related Rights Regulations 2003 (SI No. 2498).

Contents

List of Illustrations		vi
Preface		vii
	Introduction: On Questioning Blindness and What the Blind 'See'	1
1.	'Seeing with the Hands': Descartes, Blindness, and Vision	21
2.	'Suppose a man born blind...': Cubes and Spheres, Hands and Eyes	33
3.	Objects that 'touch'd his eyes': Surgical Experiments in the Recovery of Vision	57
4.	Voltaire, Buffon, and Blindness in France	85
5.	The Testimony of Blind Men: Diderot's *Lettre*	109
6.	Reading with the Fingers: Tactile Signs and the Possibilities for a Language of Touch	138
7.	Seeing with the Tongue: Sight through Other Means	160
8.	Blindness, Empathy, and 'Feeling Seeing': Literary Accounts of Blind Experience	184
References		207
Index		222

List of Illustrations

3.1 Instruments used in cataract operations. From a 1780 edition of Johannes de Gorter's *Cirugia Expurgada*. Copyright: Wellcome Library, London.   69

3.2 A double sheet showing various ophthalmology instruments, eye growths, a cataract operation, and other eye defects. Line engraving by R. Parr, 1743–45. Copyright: Wellcome Library, London   70

3.3 Guillaume Dupuytren operating on a cataract, source unknown. Copyright: Wellcome Library, London   70

5.1 Portrait of Denis Diderot by Louis-Michel van Loo, 1767. Louvre Museum, Paris. Copyright: Wikimedia Commons   122

5.2 Nicholas Saunderson [Sanderson]. Line engraving by C. F. Fritzsch after J. Vanderbank, 1719. Copyright: Wellcome Library, London   123

6.1 An illustration of competing tactile writing systems. From Merry (1937), 'Fingers for eyes', p. 275. Reprinted with permission from AAAS.   151

6.2 Standard English Braille, illustration from Merry (1937), 'Fingers for eyes', p. 276. Reprinted with permission from AAAS.   152

7.1 An early incarnation of Bach-y-Rita's TVSS system, with a tactile array for the abdomen. Reprinted from Bach-Y-Rita (1972) with permission from Elsevier.   169

7.2. The Brainport™ V100 so-called 'lollipop' TDU developed by Bach-y-Rita through his company Wicab. Copyright: Wicab Inc.   170

Preface

Naturally, material developed at various stages of the research for this book has been presented at talks and conferences, including a panel at the Association of American Geographers meeting in 2009. I have been fortunate enough to be invited to various talks in recent years, including in 2009 the Association of Medical Humanities at Durham University, the Centre for Medical Humanities at Hong Kong University, and the Department of Philosophy at Manchester Metropolitan University. In 2010, at the 'Geographies of Disability and Ageing' conference at the University of Lancaster, I presented some work in progress in the presence of the blind geographer Ruth Butler, who had inspired some of my earlier graduate study. In 2011 the Department of Communication at the University of Pittsburgh, 'The Afterlife of Phenomenology' seminar series at Northwestern University, and the Institute of Advanced Studies at the University of Edinburgh each invited me to present papers and generated useful questions and different perspectives.

Early material from the research for two chapters has therefore been published in different form. A selection of the arguments and literature covered in Chapter 8 appeared in a special issue on 'Blindness' in the literature journal *Mosaic: A Journal for the Interdisciplinary Study of Literature* as '"Looking on darkness, which the blind do see": blindness, empathy and feeling seeing' in 2013, and other material from the chapter was published as 'Blindness, empathy, and "feeling seeing": literary and insider accounts of blind experience', in *Emotion, Space and Society*, also in 2013. Referee comments in both cases helped to refine the arguments, and one suggestion in particular opened up a relevant avenue within disability studies that significantly aided the final material. Likewise, some material on sensory substitution technologies for Chapter 7 was included as part of a chapter taking a different philosophical pathway, co-written with Mazviita Chirimuuta, and published as 'A methodological Molyneux question: sensory substitution, plasticity and the unification of perceptual theory', in D. Stokes, M. Matthen, and S. Biggs (eds), *Perception and its Modalities* (Oxford: Oxford University Press, 2014).

The gestation of this project was unusually long, from initial conversations with Iain Hamilton Grant in my first academic job at the University of the West of England, to parts of it being written at the University of Exeter, and the text really coming together in my present position at the University of Pittsburgh. The project has therefore survived moves of houses, jobs, and continents. Thanks to Dhara Patel at EUP for saving the project, and my sanity, by giving it a great home at the Press. The timing was impeccable, and her enthusiasm and efficiency is appreciated.

My family have been a source of constant and unwavering support, despite all those upheavals. Thanks go to my wife, Mazviita, who diligently read and provided useful comments on drafts of all the chapters, and whose own scholarship has been an inspiration. Tinashe and Tendai were both born during the writing of the book, Tinashe near the beginning and Tendai towards the end, and have provided much joy and necessary grounding. My thanks also to my father, David, whose belief in me has been constant, even when other aspects of my work and life were not.

Introduction

On Questioning Blindness and What the Blind 'See'

The question of blindness in philosophy is never merely a question of perception. Nor, despite a perennial fascination on the part of the sighted, is it simply to ask what the blind supposedly 'see'. In the past few years, philosophy has rediscovered the senses and their modalities, but the approach usually involves adopting a rigorous scientific framework and sifting neuroscientific data in order to better understand the principles behind the processes of perception. While the neuroscience of blindness and vision is rapidly developing, and some studies are referenced in this book, there is a much longer historical dialogue between philosophy, medicine, and literature regarding the questioning of blindness, vision, and touch. Within the history of philosophy, for example, questions of blindness periodically bob and weave around, but are rarely central to, core theories or mainstream philosophical debates. And yet, as this book demonstrates, at several key junctures blindness has been used as a pre-psychological thought experiment for sighted philosophers to ask epistemological questions, to determine how we can know the world and its objects through the senses. One of the architects of that grand Enlightenment project the *Encyclopédie*, Denis Diderot, actually interviewed blind subjects at length to derive a more humanistic understanding of what the blind actually 'saw'. Subsequently, the twentieth century produced a plethora of blind and vision-impaired writers, philosophers, and psychologists who now had the means to articulate their experience in their own words, without the need for sighted authorities or intermediaries. Broadly speaking, the interrogation of blindness since Descartes' essay *Dioptrique* ('On optics', 1637) has been an inquiry by the sighted philosopher into the mechanisms of vision, but equally into the relationship between visual clarity and epistemological certainty. At one point Descartes invokes the hypothetical example of a blind man using a cane to help him navigate, proclaiming 'one might almost say that they see with their hands' (1965: 67). This is a passing observation that progressively unfolds into an epistemological interrogation, as we shall see.

Over the last few centuries, the questioning concerning blindness has become more variegated and diffuse, shifting from concerns about perception in general, but also correspondingly moving on from the unproblematised and fixed category of 'blindness' to address more specific points on the continuum of visual ability, from either congenital or acquired lack of light perception (No Light Perception or NLP) to various shades or levels of vision impairment. In this way, tracing the ongoing morphology of the questioning and categorisations of blindness, over time, helps to contextualise the historical formations and assumptions that have forged current attitudes towards blindness and sight loss. When, in his *Lettre sur les aveugles, á l'usage de ceux qui voient* ['Letter on the blind for the benefit of those who see'] (1749), Diderot marvels at the calculating tables invented and used by a blind professor of mathematics, or exhorts his readers to share the wonder of a blind Frenchman's articulation of a philosophical worldview, the modern reader recognises this style of presentation, over two hundred and fifty years later, of the cognitively capable yet introspective blind subject. As the historical narrative of this book unfolds, it will become increasingly clear that such tropes of blindness are at once startlingly modern – in the way they deal with a certain form of subjectivity, the blind subject – but also historically confining and pervasive, as we grasp to what extent we owe a key historical period of philosophical, literary, and medical inquiry the sighted reader's understanding of blindness, and the somewhat sensational fascination with what the blind supposedly 'see'.

Within this broad interrogation of blindness, in each of the following chapters we look to distinct historical time periods in order to distil key conceptual questions that had currency within, and beyond, philosophy at that time. Such questions include: what is the relationship between touch and vision, and on what basis might we recognise an object through touch if we have never seen it? How can sensations in one modality can be translated into another modality, say from touch to vision? How can forms of tactile literacy premised on cross-modal perception open up a world of literature, science, and even cartography to a blind reader? What do the blind perceive immediately after cataract surgery, and how do they subsequently learn rules about perspective and perform spatial judgements over time? How do sensory prostheses enhance perception for those without sight through technologies of sensory substitution, where tactile or auditory sense-data stand in for vision, thereby calling into question what 'seeing' actually is? And, when countenancing one's own impending blindness due to disease or age, what kinds of emotional responses and empathic mechanisms are in play? In posing a series of questions about blindness we are not adhering to a particular philosophical school or tradition, but painting a broader historical picture of a dialogue between philosophy and blindness, of how blindness has been conceived in relation to touch and vision. We chart how particular debates, correspondences, and investigations between philosophers, initially in Britain and France, came to influence not only early psychological investigations, but also contemporary attitudes to the blind by the sighted. While none of this book is written in a way that purposefully privileges a sighted reader, it is nonetheless important to acknowledge that the majority of early inquiries into blindness were pursued by sighted individuals, including scientists, philosophers, and surgeons, and so their questioning of blindness in general, or of particular blind individuals, is inevitably posed in terms of 'seeing'.

To pose any form of 'question' or inquiry into blindness, to subject blindness (or the blind subject) to questioning, is always inevitably to counterpose the question of vision, of what 'seeing' supposedly consists in. To what extent any such questions are potentially derived from an overarching humanistic inquiry into what the blind 'see' is at once uncomfortable and unavoidable. If sighted readers see blindness and the process of becoming blind as a projection of their own fears, say, then we acknowledge an inherent asymmetry within this enterprise. Remember, 'for the benefit of those who see' is the subtitle of Diderot's essay on blindness. As is argued in more detail below, we might question the nature of the sighted subject's empathic response. Descartes considering a hypothetical blind man in *Dioptrique* in 1637, Molyneux posing a question about blindness to John Locke in 1688, Diderot interviewing a blind man outside Paris in 1749, or Brian Magee corresponding with the blind philosopher Martin Milligan in 1998, each in their own way betrays a recurring motif, the sighted philosopher questioning the blind subject ostensibly to discern something of the 'truth' of the experience of blindness. The sighted reader's perennial fascination with what the blind 'see' was the subject of an essay in 2003 by Oliver Sacks in *The New Yorker*, although Sacks's instantiation, being relatively recent, drew criticism from blind and vision-impaired respondents (for a thoughtful critical essay see Candela 2003). The historical interrogation of 'blindness' (and more precise definitions and sub-categories of that term will follow shortly) is consequently irreducible to any monothematic or cohesive 'question' concerning vision or 'seeing' that might emerge, in differing forms, across various time periods. Only by acknowledging the entangled relation between these too broad labels 'blindness' and 'vision', which can be broken down according to a more granular spectrum of the physiological specificities of the mechanisms of sight, vision impairment, or total lack of light perception, can we proceed further in the questioning of blindness. As this historical narrative unfolds through each chapter, the questioning therefore necessarily involves an awareness of such entanglement, and consequently decries any broad categorisation of 'blindness' and 'vision'. Inevitably, however, any sustained motif concerning blindness and its treatment by sighted individuals and publics simply cannot escape accusations of an asymmetric voyeurism, a fascination with 'the' experience of blindness. In this we might follow alongside Garland-Thomson's investigation of disability, 'The politics of staring', where the encounter with images of the disabled body is fraught with 'a tangle of distance, anxiety and identification' (2002: 57).

Therefore, the term 'blindness' in this text is employed in as specific a sense as possible. Unfortunately, until the latter part of the twentieth century, records or descriptions of blind individuals remained a largely undifferentiated category, where the breakdown into types, origins, or levels of visual ability were simply unknown, unrecorded, or inconsistent. Current employment of the term 'blindness' involves the legal definition according to the World Health Organization. Within our current historical era of medicalised late capitalism, then, the sighted should technically be more aware of the multiple causes of visual impairment, and the differences in visual ability of non-sighted or visually impaired populations. As such, the variation in visual ability within what is categorised by legal and medical communities as 'blindness' underlines the fact that for each label of 'blind', NLP, or low vision there remains, even within that category, a spectrum of visual ability. For example, with an advanced case of the inherited degenerative eye disease retinitis pigmentosa, the artist Andrew Potok found some residual vision remained. Providing the uninitiated sighted reader with a beautifully descriptive passage that conveys something of the patchwork of his visual experience, he clarifies that 'blindness isn't blackness':

> My field now, piecing together the odd bits here and there, is less than 5 degrees. Because the losses are a patchwork of dead or dying cells, my functional vision is difficult to understand. [...] In the full

mosaic of cells, the dysfunctional ones are not black, nor are there sharp boundaries between them and the neighboring useful cells. Blindness isn't blackness; it is nothingness. I have, therefore, on my retina, a tiny amount of somethingness surrounded and influenced by a vast nothingness. There is a disorganization of the whole; everything is ill-fitting, jagged and incomplete. [...] Objects appear or vanish abruptly and inexplicably. Nothing makes spatial sense, so I put together visual cues based largely on memory and imagination. For me, perceived reality is spotty, appearing in a kind of charged, flickering motion. (Potok 2007: 35–6)

Further rich descriptions of experiences of blindness, and of the sighted writer anticipating and then undergoing the process of becoming blind, feature in subsequent chapters. For now, we consider how we have historically come to understand blindness, and especially blindness as darkness, in the first place. This works as an opportunity to provide an introductory overview for the reader of some pertinent historical-philosophical 'moments', that is, articulations of blindness, vision, and touch through medical, philosophical, literary, and public discourses that engaged the imagination and stimulated inquiry at that juncture. One of the earliest and most productive of such moments, unsurprisingly, is the Enlightenment.

Blindness in the age of Enlightenment

Foucault's great contribution in *L'Archéologie du savoir* ['The archaeology of knowledge'] (1969) was to outline how a whole chaos of signs enters into a universal regime of systems of representation, what he calls an 'episteme', which historically govern and structure the bounds of what can be known. It is not knowledge (*connaissance*) as such, although episteme is of course the Greek root of epistemology. An episteme is 'something like a world-view' (Foucault 2002: 211), a prevailing mode of knowledge and investigation, what makes it possible for a discourse to be taken as 'knowledge' and then as less disputable scientific 'fact'. But an episteme is not to be equated with 'knowledge' itself. To discern an episteme is to recognise the orderly 'unconscious' structures underlying the production of scientific knowledge in a particular time and place. The episteme does not explain how fixed branches of knowledge (*connaissance*) came into being, but 'the total set of relations that unite, at a given period, the discursive practices that give rise to epistemological figures, sciences, and possibly formalized systems' wherein each of these 'discursive formations' (2002: 211) allows the formalisation into distinct approaches to knowledge or inquiry. It is not a fixed explanation for how these approaches to knowledge came about, as these are continually morphing and being reshaped; but an episteme acknowledges this since 'it is a constantly moving set of articulations, shifts and coincidences that are established, only to give rise to others' (2002: 211). Something like a worldview, then, or comparable to Thomas Kuhn's analysis of scientific revolutions as shifting 'paradigms', the episteme applies not only to scientific frameworks but also to other human endeavours or modes of inquiry. Foucault gives the example of the biology and psychology of sexuality in the wake of Freud, which is not reducible to a 'science' of sex per se. Posing such questions led to far-reaching effects, with coruscating shifts in attitudes and institutions.

There is no such straightforward parallel in terms of blindness. However, what we might understand, on the one hand, as a provocation in the form of a philosophical question and, on the other, as a guiding myth for understanding a certain stage of intellectual history is a philosophical moment concerning blindness which does indeed cut across a series of disciplinary and institutional boundaries, throwing up in its wake speculative answers throughout Europe and encouraging the gathering of early empirical evidence for a definitive answer, an answer that never quite arrived. This was the Molyneux question, first articulated in a letter to the philosopher John Locke by the Irishman William Molyneux in 1688. If not exactly an episteme, this particular question essentially reframes the perennial question about what the blind 'see' to ask hypothetically what the blind *would* see were their vision suddenly to be restored:

> Suppose a man born blind, and now adult, and taught by his touch to distinguish between a cube and a sphere of the same metal, and nighly of the same bigness, so as to tell, when he felt one and the other, which is the cube, which the sphere. Suppose then the cube and sphere placed on a table, and the blind man be made to see: *quaere*, whether *by his sight before he touched them*, he could now distinguish and tell which is the globe, which the cube? (*Essay* II.IX.8)

Molyneux's letter is paraphrased in the second edition of Locke's *An Essay Concerning Human Understanding* (1692), and is then followed by Locke's answer:

> I agree with this thinking gentleman, whom I am proud to call my friend, in his answer to this problem; and am of opinion that the blind man, at first sight, would not be able with certainty to say which was

the globe, which the cube, whilst he only saw them; though he could unerringly name them by his touch, and certainly distinguish them by the difference of their figures felt. (*Essay* II.IX.8)

While seemingly innocuous, Molyneux's question soon unleashed a whole nested series of concerns within philosophy about innate knowledge and the value of experience, and, through Voltaire, helped overturn the established philosophical doctrine in France of rationalism, exemplified in the writing of Descartes. Over successive decades, Molyneux's provocative question encouraged a turn to empiricism and what Alain Grosrichard terms a 'prescientific psychology' (2012: 210), reaching out to scientific verification through early evidence after cataract operations, most famously by the surgeon William Cheselden in his report to the Royal Society of 1728. Unfolding across the centuries it continues to be debated in terms of neonatal psychology and recent neuroscience (e.g. Held et al. 2011). Its answer concerns blindness, more specifically the man born blind (*l'aveugle-né*) who is restored to sight through an operation (*l'aveugle-operé*). As a motif, or the instantiation of an episteme, it refers beyond mere historical facticity or surgical possibility to encapsulate a wider intellectual concern of the culture at the time about the relationship between vision and truth, and correspondingly between blindness and knowledge. In his earlier *Naissance de la clinique* ['The birth of the clinic'] (1963), Foucault outlines the discursive power of this combination at this historical juncture:

> What allows man to resume contact with childhood and to rediscover the permanent birth of truth is this bright, distant, open naïvety of the gaze. Hence the two great mythical experiences on which the philosophy of the eighteenth century had wished to base its beginning: the foreign spectator in an unknown country, and the man born blind restored to light. (2003: 78)

The concern with the man born blind (*l'aveugle-né*), and its uptake not only by certain philosophers but perennially by a wider sighted public, will indeed demonstrate the discursive power of myth, yet permits a series of philosophical questions that delineate the terms and boundaries of a pre-scientific psychology for at least eight decades after Molyneux. The public interest was only compounded and accelerated through the series of accounts of *aveugles-operé* by surgeons in the wake of Cheselden, such as those of Joseph Hillmer and Jacques Daviel in 1748.

The Molyneux question is pivotal and, while hypothetical in its original form, explicitly instantiates the Foucauldian mythical experience of the 'man born blind restored to light'. Indeed, developing Foucault's point further, this was '*a new kind of experiment*' (Grosrichard 2012: 210, his emphasis) since, for reasons that will become clear, it was not simply matching a theoretical hypothesis with an experimental verification, as a psychological experiment might do. Instead, Grosrichard is employing the double meaning in French of *expérience*, as both scientific or thought 'experiment', but also 'experience' as we commonly understand it. Thus, for Grosrichard, the most significant fallout of the Molyneux question is not this eighteenth-century psychological experiment considered 'as a verification of speculative hypotheses', which is how the question is historically understood; instead, argues Grosrichard, its impact lies in being 'an experiment of prescientific psychology invented by the philosopher in order to replace another kind of experiment, an experiment or experience of philosophy – one invented *by empiricist and sensualist philosophy* so as to maintain the coherence of its discourse' (2012: 210, his emphasis). The import of the Molyneux question for philosophy and early psychology therefore lies in its being a positively disruptive force that considers the senses and their modalities in a more sophisticated way than before. What results is an enriched empiricism, in Britain and then France, that dislodges the vestiges of dogmatic rationalism within science. For example Voltaire, in popularising the Molyneux question and Cheselden's surgery through importing British ideas into France, wrote in his *Éléments de la philosophie de Newton* (1738) of the impact of the new British empiricism for the hitherto entrenched Cartesianism of the scientists in his native land. Voltaire's recounting of the Molyneux question and Cheselden's ocular surgery had clearly drawn the attention of other sensationist philosophers, but in a manner consistent with Foucault's identification of 'the man born blind restored to light', as a rediscovery of 'the permanent birth of truth' through the 'bright, distant, open naivety of the gaze' (Foucault 2003: 78).

Despite the Molyneux question being pitted in 1692, the mythical aspect remained and evidence was lacking or inconclusive. La Mettrie, in his *Histoire naturelle de l'âme* ['Treatise of the soul'] (1745), and then Condillac in his *Essai sur l'origine des connaisances humaines* ['Essay on the origin of human knowledge'] (1746), were wise to this, critiquing available data and judging the partiality of Cheselden's experiment. 'By dint of tormenting the newly sighted man,' wrote La Mettrie, 'they got him to say what they wanted to hear' (in Weygand 2009: 60). What 'they', the Enlightenment philosophers, scientists, and assorted men of letters actually wanted to hear, of course, was what best fitted their adopted philosophical frameworks, as the following chapters will reveal. At its core, however, the naivety involved in the trope of the blind gaze being newly restored to sight remained unchallenged, and it was not until Diderot's *Lettre sur les aveugles* of 1749 that blindness became sufficiently demystified for the idea to gain acceptance that the 'common' blind were not in fact intellectually or spiritually inferior.

At this stage it would be useful to establish a distinction between two forms of blindness: first, a 'hypothetical' form that lies at a certain level of abstraction, characteristic of the questioning of the blind subject by the sighted, and which assumes a monothematic truth to blindness and therefore permits inquiry into a distinctive, generic form of 'blind' experience; secondly, what we might term the 'actual' medical-legal form of blindness that admits of a number of causes, including congenital disease, acquired blindness through accident or preventable disease, and consequently a spectrum of abilities and visual acuities within the encompassing label of 'blindness'.

'Hypothetical' blindness

> Visual culture entails a meditation on blindness, the invisible, the unseen, the unseeable, and the overlooked. (Mitchell 2002: 170)

To question blindness is to question what seeing, and sighted experience, entails. One of the more pervasive figurations of blindness by the sighted occurs as an 'empty form', a 'Hypothetical Blind Man' (Kleege 2005: 180), a blank-blind figure upon which speculative epistemologies, or the anxieties of the sighted, are projected. As opposed to interrogating the subject of blindness, then, often an unnamed blind subject stands in for an area of inquiry, an idea, an anxiety, and consequently this reflects a cultural attitude to 'blindness' that has been historically persistent. Although the 'hypothetical blind man' was coined by Gitter (2001), the blind academic Georgina Kleege recognises this phenomenon in its capitalised form to emphasise its generic status. This hypothetical figure is used as 'a prop for theories of consciousness', since:

> He is the patient subject of endless thought experiments where the experience of the world through four senses can be compared to the experience of the world through five. He is asked to describe his

understanding of specific visual phenomena – perspective, reflection, refraction, color, form recognition – as well as visual aids and enhancements – mirrors, lenses, telescopes, microscopes. (Kleege 2005: 180)

The historical-philosophical moment of questioning blindness, after Molyneux, was consequently not simply a return to any pure or monolithic experience of being blind per se. The somewhat enriched hypothetical exercise or thought experiment involves an almost empathic placement of the reader, such that the reader must put her or himself '*in the place* of the originary psychological subject' under question, in Grosrichard's words (2012: 211, his emphasis). The thought experiment of Molyneux's question prompts an extended consideration of the *expérience* of blindness and the blind man made to see. This placement of the inquirer or interrogator into blindness is present even in the wording of the question. For the wording of Molyneux's question highlights the imperative for the philosopher to place himself in the position of the *aveugle-né*: 'Suppose a man born blind...' says Locke, after all. As such, the hypothetical blind subject functions, thinks Grosrichard, as an 'instrument of experimentation or experience' [*expérience*], and like Gitter and Kleege, the questioner therefore imposes an 'empty form' (2012: 213) or a marked place for the subject to consider blindness and the 'truth' of seeing. Whether for the purposes of fulfilling the curiosity of a sighted reader, or for exploring an epistemological question about the senses of touch and sight, this movement to an 'empty form' is to return to a hypothetical, generic blind subject, the blank-blind figure.

Putting Locke's formulation of Molyneux's question to a hypothetical blind man would therefore be predictable and unenlightening. For 'he was, after all, only the crude realization of the pure blind man posited by Molyneux' (Grosrichard 2012: 214). The 'pure blind man', the empty form, was invoked as a hypothetical construct in part so that the authority of the sighted interrogator was maintained over the blind subject, and also as a living illustration of the role of the senses, especially sight and touch, in the production of knowledge. Even Cheselden's account of his cataract operation concerned an unnamed thirteen-year-old boy, with minimal articulation of the experience through the boy's own words.

Given the supposition, or indeed superposition, between sighted reader-philosopher and *aveugle-né* in Locke's formulation of Molyneux's problem, we should acknowledge that empathic entanglement works in both directions. Another major waypoint in the philosophical interrogation of blindness, Diderot's *Lettre sur les aveugles*, encourages an alternative approach to Locke: not to make the philosopher-reader take the place of the blind subject, but rather the promise of enabling the blind to articulate the truth of their experience, effectively turning them into philosophers, that is, 'thoroughly aware of the gaps in [their] experience and master of [their] language' (Grosrichard 2012: 218). Reversing Molyneux's imperative to philosophers to make themselves blind, to hypothesise an empty form of the *aveugle-né*, then, the multiple subjects of Diderot's 'experiment' in the *Lettre* are a series of actual, living, blind men, with the suggestion of direct contact and interaction with them. Each was educated enough to be a 'philosopher', that is, having a certain standard of learning and education, in order to claim authority over their own experience. This was important for Diderot, as only then could they articulate in everyday language those elements of experience that are 'missing' or lost, what differentiates them from the perception of the point of reference, what Garland-Thomson (1997) terms the 'normate', sighted, subject. After Molyneux's question, Diderot's *Lettre* is assuredly a step in the right direction, but the authority of the text overall was compromised. As we shall see, his portrayal of the experiences and views of his blind interlocutors was questionable, and the voicing of Diderot's own religious views through the purported deathbed confession of a blind professor was, after publication, literally scandalous. If the *aveugle-né* furnished philosophy during Locke's time with a malleable example, the blank-blind subject or 'empty form', this was yet to be verified through ocular surgery. Yet, since the authority of later medical reports of actual ocular surgery failed to answer the hypothetical questions definitively, even the beneficiaries of ocular surgery were not free from compromised authority, from adopting the views of the interrogator, of being unwittingly involved in fabrication. 'It is up to philosophy entirely to invent its experimentation, to *fabricate* its blind man', as Grosrichard observes (2012: 219, his emphasis). Nevertheless, it remains surprising just how long it took for the interrogation of 'blindness', in the wake of Cheselden's report and of Diderot's interviews with learned blind men, to depart from such fabrication and achieve more detailed and involved testimony, in their own words, from blind subjects about the truth of their actual experience.

'Actual' blindness: on blindness, 'blindness', and vision impairment

Moving away from sighted philosophers as the arbiters of significance for the various forms of blindness and blind experience, first-person authoritative published accounts of blindness, and of the process of becoming blind, have been popular since Thérèse-Adèle Husson in 1825, and of course Helen Keller's autobiographies, the first of which was published in 1903. But here we make important terminological caveats. The distinction between 'blindness' and 'vision impairment' is crucial in both medical science and social history, and there is something of an inexact continuum between the two states. Neurologically and physiologically, 'blindness' can refer to a dysfunction of the visual cortex (cortical blindness) occurring from congenital defect or disease, or from later accidental brain injury, or damage to optic nerve or eye tissue, for example. Ophthalmological and legal definitions of blindness focus on the ability to perceive light, colours, and shapes, such that 'total' blindness is equated with the complete absence of sensitivity to light, denoted as No Light Perception (NLP), whereas some light perception is indicative of residual vision, and therefore of severe vision impairment. According to various governmental and institutional scales there are few cases of NLP, and most of those classified as blind have measurably severe forms of vision impairment. In most countries, including the UK and the US, assessments of blindness or the level of vision impairment are based on World Health Organization classifications of the ability to see over prescribed distances without forms of optical correction such as spectacles. The standard measure for perfect eyesight is '20/20', referring to the distance in feet from which a person with naturally good visual acuity can reliably distinguish a pair of objects. This is a measure of visual acuity. With 20/200 visual acuity, the state of being technically legally blind in the US, for example, an individual would have to stand 20 feet from an object to see it with the same degree of clarity as a normally sighted person could from 200 feet. Approximately 10 per cent of those deemed legally blind, by any measure, have no vision. The rest have some vision, from minimal light perception alone to relatively good acuity. 'Low vision' is sometimes used to describe visual acuities from 20/70 to 20/200, according to the American Foundation for the Blind (AFB 2002). Visual acuity is only one measure of blindness or vision impairment, since a restricted visual field is also a factor. Tunnel vision, a restriction in peripheral vision, negatively affects the visual field and an individual's situational awareness. Again, a restricted peripheral range can be measured against a norm or standard of 180 degrees, and a field limited to 20 degrees would suggest blindness. This set of explanations surrounding legal and medical definitions of 'blindness' and vision impairment is relatively neat, but promises a consistency in usage that will be impossible to maintain when examining the rather inexact previous historical and philosophical deployments of the term.

This shading of abilities within blindness is itself aggravated by factors such as whether the vision loss is congenital, so that the subject has never had exposure to visual aspects of shape, perspective, or colour, or whether the blindness is acquired, in which case the subject has been exposed to those prior visual experiences. If acquired, further considerations are the speed of onset, whether sudden through accident or injury, or more gradually through irreversible factors such as ophthalmic disease, vitamin B deficiency (especially in impoverished populations), or by the onset of age which alters our visual abilities over time. According to the National Institute of Health (NIH) in the United States, and the World Health Organization, cataracts are the leading cause of blindness in the world, responsible for 51 per cent of the world's blind population (WHO 2010: 3). Cataracts are usually either prenatal or occur in later life, starting with a fogging of vision as a result of a change of opacity in the lens. At least in those countries where healthcare is accessible, cataracts are easily operable. The cloudy lens is removed through an incision in the cornea, the thin transparent front of the eye, and replaced with an artificial one. An astonishing fact is that, by the age of eighty, 'more than half of all people in the United States either will have a cataract or have had cataract surgery' (NIH 2008: 14).

Other causes of blindness are not so easily treated. Glaucoma is in second place globally as a cause of blindness, resulting from irreversible damage to the optic nerve, and then the retina, through intraocular pressure from the aqueous humours. This pressure build-up is slow, and changes to the visual field are so gradual that sight loss occurs almost imperceptibly. Damage to the optic nerve leads to small blind spots in the visual field known as scotoma, and if left untreated these increase in size and conjoin so that only tunnel vision remains (Hollins 1989: 16). The third largest cause of blindness is age-related macular degeneration (AMD). The macula is the central part of the retina with the greatest density of cones, and is therefore responsible for the highest visual acuity. The macula is involved in seeing fine detail for the performance of such activities as reading or sewing.

If, after Descartes, and with some poetic licence, we consider the eyes to be analogous to the hands, then the macula is the hand. The fovea, a small pit within the macula with an even denser distribution of photoreceptors (rods and cones), would be the fingertips. The macula is susceptible to damage through age and toxic substances.

Further causes of blindness include retinitis pigmentosa (RP), the hereditary condition that the painter Potok wrote of above, whereby a progressive loss of function of photoreceptors on the retina leads to tunnel vision and eventually total vision loss. Trachoma is caused by a disease prevalent in underdeveloped parts of the world, transmitted by flies, and is preventable. However, if trachoma is correlated with those parts of the world that suffer extreme poverty, another cause of blindness on the WHO watchlist is exactly the opposite. Diabetic retinopathy is equally preventable, and results from failure to inject insulin as directed by a doctor, leading to changes in retinal blood circulation which then damage the retina. Diabetic populations are on the increase in advanced industrial economies like the US and the UK. Ninety per cent of global diabetes is Type II diabetes, which has some genetic aspect but which is mostly a result of obesity and high blood sugar. Hence, whether poverty and disease on the one hand, or excess of calories in consumer economies on the other, the causes of the vast majority of blindness around the world are preventable, given equitable access to healthcare and resources. The WHO estimates that, globally, '80% of visual impairment can be prevented or cured' (WHO 2012). Given such diversity in global causes of blindness, and the various definitions of 'blindness' and 'vision impairment', we also acknowledge the variability of visual abilities over time as populations age. With large-scale demographic shifts towards older populations in advanced industrial economies, the number of older people requiring ophthalmic intervention will only increase.

Nonetheless, everyday usage of the word 'blindness' for the sighted reader stubbornly proffers a particular imaginary of a non-sighted other: 'the blind'. As Georgina Kleege points out: 'Of course, it's the word *blind* that causes all the problems. To most people blindness means total, absolute darkness, a complete absence of any visual experience', yet 'only about 10 per cent of the legally blind have this degree of impairment' (1999: 14, original emphasis). Likewise, the Scottish writer Candia McWilliam evinces a similar unease with conventional understandings of blindness as blackness (and therefore NLP):

> Blindness, and I gather that this is so for many who cannot see, is not a solid or unmodulated blackness such as one might imagine comes

over the head of a hawk when you put on its hood. In addition my blindness could be termed illegitimate, since it is not so that my eyes cannot see. (2010: 4–5)

The way we deploy 'blindness' in everyday linguistic usage is similarly revealing. In a dictionary with thirteen entries under 'blindness', only one refers directly to the actual medical definition. The rest are a mixture of metaphors, including such negative affects as 'blind fear' and 'blind rage', deployed as literary tropes. The remaining definitions, argues Bolt, display connotations that are 'split between ignorance and concealment' (2003: 519), commonly involving *lack*. Blind ignorance (lacking knowledge), blind stupor (lacking awareness), blind prejudice (lacking a critical or questioning attitude), blind taste test (tasting without looking), blind presentation (lacking preparation or information): such negative connotations reveal a configuration of readerly empathy, where blindness as darkness is similarly understood as lack (of light), as deprivation. As Julia Rodas articulates, such casual connotations of blindness may not be innocent metaphors, as such, but involve a metonymic relation. In other words, when we speak of 'blindness' we might mean something different:

> The wealth of meaning that has been fabricated around the idea of blindness, our cultural reliance on blindness as metaphor, thus metonymizes the blind man, recreating him as a figure of speech, the component of a joke, a poem; or the same gesture allows us, blind or sighted, to recreate ourselves as metaphorically blind. (2009: 117)

Conversely, any attempt at the articulation and redescription of experiences of blindness by blind authors such as Kleege, Hull, or Torey (pursued in detail in chapter 8), or of the anxieties of those actually facing up to becoming blind, might be welcomed as a corrective to the awkward and asymmetrical mapping of sighted readerly empathy over the construct of 'blindness'.

Overview of the chapters

Having revealed points of significance in the overall landscape of the book, here I offer a chapter-by-chapter overview.

The first chapter ' "Seeing with the Hands": Descartes, Blindness, and Vision' sets up the framework for understanding and validating non-visual experiences by introducing one of the earliest tangential philosophical engagements with blindness in Descartes' famous essay *Dioptrique* ('On optics', 1637). As part of an explanation for the mechanisms of light hitting the retina, he makes the analogy of a hypothetical blind man walking with a stick. Further analogies between hands and eyes are explicitly referenced and developed later by Diderot and Voltaire. This chapter examines some philosophical and psychological assumptions behind the analogy, involving the possibility of transfer from one sensory modality (vision) to another (touch). Raising this still-contested question at this early stage of the book lays the groundwork for the thought experiments and medical findings discussed in succeeding chapters, and the kinds of technologies designed to aid the blind and vision-impaired such as sensory substitution technology. Descartes' initial analogy therefore neatly solidifies an influential conceptualisation of blindness for several centuries, initiating a philosophical relation between blindness, vision, and touch that will be developed and problematised in England, then in France, and which affects the development of early psychology.

The second chapter, ' "Suppose a man born blind…": Cubes and Spheres, Hands and Eyes', takes up the story a few decades after Descartes' initial philosophical speculations, leading up to the more refined question concerning cross-modal perception that Molyneux was to ask. The reason Ernst Cassirer called it *'the* central question of eighteenth century epistemology and psychology' in 1951 is the crux of this chapter. The context and set-up to Locke's treatment of visual knowledge as 'Understanding' in Book II of the *Essay* reveals a mechanism for how sensations become knowledge ('objects of Understanding'), and Locke illustrates this by way of a camera obscura, the darkened room. An epistemological model based on darkness and light is productive for thinking about blindness and seeing, as it leads into discussion by Locke of the Molyneux correspondence, along with other mentions of blindness in the *Essay*. Having posed the Molyneux question, therefore, this chapter first examines the continuity with the previous chapter's Cartesian analogy between hands and eyes, and secondly explores responses by contemporaries and near contemporaries, especially Berkeley's *An Essay Towards a New Theory of Vision* (1709), written directly as a response to Locke, and Voltaire's popularisation of the problem in France a few decades later, and Buffon's and Reid's response.

'Objects that "touch'd his eyes": Surgical Experiments in the Recovery of Vision' is the third chapter. While philosophically inclined speculation was rife in the common rooms and parlours of the eighteenth century, surgical techniques soon caught up with philosophical discussion and began to offer more concrete evidence. William Cheselden's cataract surgery and report to the Royal Society in 1728 caused a surge of public interest in the dramatic realisation, after bandages are removed, of what the formerly blind now 'see'. The importance of this for Molyneux's question is clear: now subjects with prolonged experience of blindness could answer the question directly. At first sight, literally, Cheselden reports the young blind patient saying 'he thought all Objects whatever touch'd his Eyes' (1728: 448). Despite the rarity of such operations, the insights into the visual system, the process of seeing and learning to see, and its interaction with other senses are invaluable. For these newly sighted subjects spatial perception, especially depth and perspective, are initially problematic, leading to the appreciation that the visual system works in accordance with the other senses and movement, as opposed to raw 'sight' or purely optical information. A history of such surgical experiments is offered in this chapter, with accounts from popular magazines like *Tatler* about the oculist Roger Grant, along with Cheselden's more scientific report to the Royal Society, and the work of twentieth-century psychologist Alberto Valvo. But the chapter is bookended by a famous 1963 case study in the psychology of perception, Richard Gregory's patient 'S.B.' who, in Gregory's words, 'learned how to see' after an operation to restore his vision, but thereafter retreated into his familiar world of darkness.

The fourth chapter is 'Voltaire, Buffon, and Blindness in France'. If the issues raised around blindness for Descartes, Locke, and Berkeley originated in philosophical inquiry and speculative epistemology, and the results of surgical intervention lay within scientific experimentation, the subsequent uptake of these ideas, the influence of Locke's empiricism as a challenge to the entrenched rationalism of Cartesianism in Europe, and a new emphasis on the centrality of experience and sensation was kick-started by Voltaire in exile and developed into a fully fledged sensationalism through Condillac. It is some measure of the significance of the Molyneux question, thinks Ernst Cassirer, that it continued to stimulate responses in France several decades later: Voltaire in his *Élements de la philosophie de Newton* (1738) offered 'an extensive exposition of the problem', and Condillac even 'declares that it contains the source and key to all modern psychology' (1979: 109). Cheselden's 1728 report provided further stimulus to the intellectual imagination. After Voltaire introduced an enthusiastic French readership to Molyneux's question and Cheselden's case study, there followed intense interest in blindness on the part of La Mettrie, Condillac, Diderot, and Buffon.

The contributions of French commentators in the wake of these new scientific discoveries is the concern of this chapter, concentrating on Voltaire's popular introduction of the Molyneux problem and Buffon's placing of blindness and vision within the larger explanatory framework of the monumental *Histoire naturelle* (1749), his influential multi-volume work. To illustrate his ideas Buffon considers a hypothetical neonate who must correlate hands with eyes in order to see; the hand is 'constantly measuring' so that distance and perspective can be learned, implying that the blind still have spatial concepts.

'The Testimony of Blind Men: Diderot's *Lettre*' is the fifth chapter. In 1749 Diderot composed his celebrated *Lettre sur les aveugles*, which dealt directly with blindness and what the blind supposedly 'see'. Rather than treating the issue as an amusing parlour game, or using public performances of ocular surgery to fuel philosophical speculation, Diderot instead sought out the testimony of an actual blind man in the French town of Puiseaux. Referring back to Molyneux's question, and having considered Cheselden's postoperative evidence, Diderot's contribution here is a multi-stranded essay that includes the marriage of blind testimony of spatial perception to now-familiar philosophical issues, suggests possible ways of communicating through touching on the skin, and scandalously attributes an atheist disquisition to the deathbed confessions of the blind English mathematician Nicholas Saunderson. Nevertheless, in suggesting a 'clear and precise language of touch' (1916a: 90) he would prefigure the development of embossed scripts for the blind, and eventually the systematic characters of Braille a century later. Diderot's account of Saunderson, Lucasian Professor of Mathematics at Cambridge, who although blind could perform complex calculations through the use of pins on a board, demonstrates how touching equates to 'visualising' numbers and an increased tactile acuity as a result of vision loss. Diderot refers to Descartes' analogy that the blind 'see' with their hands, and his essay ends as it starts, with the consideration of Molyneux's question. While situating the detailed arguments of Diderot within the larger core argument, this chapter also considers how both Diderot's and Voltaire's treatments reiterate the popular fascination with what the blind 'see'.

The sixth chapter, 'Reading with the Fingers: Tactile Signs and the Possibilities for a Language of Touch', takes forward Diderot's plea for a tactile language for the blind. The accidental discovery by Valentin Haüy that embossed script could be read by the fingers paved the way for the concrete development of a fully fledged haptic reading system. Haüy's discovery implied that 'sensitive fingers [...] could take the place of insensitive eyes' (Farrell 1956), further cementing Descartes' analogy of hands and eyes. The story of tactile writing systems is spurred in part by shame, as a means of including the blind in literate culture. Haüy's *Essai sur l'education des aveugles* ['Essay on the education of the blind'] of 1786 summarised his purpose: 'to teach the blind reading, by the assistance of books, where the letters are rendered palpable by their elevation above the surface of the paper' (1894: 9). That touch allowed a form of reading through the skin showed a way of retrieving dignity and independence for the blind, an ethos continued through the establishment of his private school for the blind in Paris. Here the evolution of competing writing systems and their role in education and access to literature and mathematics is detailed, as Braille's system spread to other countries including Britain and the US, and was famously endorsed by Helen Keller, whose own remarkable story of reading and communicating through the skin is so compelling.

'Seeing with the Tongue: Sight through Other Means' is the seventh chapter. Descartes' discussion of the cane, the tactile calculating board of Saunderson, and tactile mapping experiments at Haüy's blind school are examples of early mechanisms that substituted touch for sight. Expanding from the formulation of Molyneux's original question about vision and touch, this chapter concerns research in the technology of sensory substitution. In the 1960s Paul Bach-y-Rita experimented with his TVSS (Tactile-Visual Sensory Substitution) devices, which transcoded optical information from a camera feed on to the surface of the tongue (Bach-y-Rita et al. 1998) and the back (Bach-y-Rita et al. 1969). This provided constantly updated low-resolution information as a means of spatial guidance for the blind. Reports of such sensory substitution demonstrate that information gleaned by one sense modality is partially translatable to another sense modality. Recent examples such as the BrainPort™ by WICAB lead to insights into the nature of 'seeing', extend the Molyneux problem into more recent technological territory, and speak to the possibilities of cross-modal perception raised throughout this book.

The eighth chapter, 'Blindness, Empathy, and "Feeling Seeing": Literary Accounts of Blind Experience', turns from treatments of blindness in philosophy in order to look at tropes and figures of blind subjects, and articulations of the process of going blind, in literature. There is a critical concern with the underlying fascination on the part of the sighted with what the blind 'see'. The idea of empathic vision, or 'feeling seeing', reveals an allied inquisitiveness concerning what the blind feel, and this is pursued through a series of authorial voices, persistent myths, and tropes. Departing from the 'hypothetical Blind Man', we focus upon what Jorge Luis Borges terms the 'pathetic moment' of his own becoming blind (1973). The twentieth century offered a number of highly personal and affecting accounts of experiences of blindness, and the process of becoming blind, and these are effectively filtered through Borges. These voices include the deaf-blind Helen Keller's *The Story of My Life* (1903) and *The World I Live In* (1908), John Hull's account of descending into 'deep' blindness in *Touching the Rock* (1991), Magee and Milligan's philosophical exchange of letters *Sight Unseen* (1998), literary theorist Georgina Kleege's similarly titled account of macular degeneration (1999), and most recently Oliver Sacks's autobiographical account of vision impairment through ocular cancer, *The Mind's Eye* (2010).

Chapter 1

'Seeing with the Hands': Descartes, Blindness, and Vision

The nobility of sight

The centrality of the eye in particular, and the visual in general, is termed 'ocularcentrism' by the intellectual historian Martin Jay in his monumental survey of French philosophical approaches to vision, *Downcast Eyes* (1994). Although his coinage was novel, it has long been understood that the legacy of Plato and Descartes led to a cultural and philosophical bias towards vision and the eye, involving the flourishing of visual metaphors and models for truth and knowledge, more than any other sense organ or modality. The ocularcentric narrative includes Aristotle's placing of sight at the apex of the hierarchy of the senses in *De anima* ('On the soul') and *De sensu et sensibilibus* ('On the senses and sensibilities'), both written around 350 BC. Likewise, Descartes' assertion at the beginning of his essay *Dioptrique* that 'sight is the most comprehensive and the noblest' of the senses (1965: 65) is one of the most representative single encapsulations of visualistic bias in philosophy, and is taken as a starting point in Hans Jonas's influential essay 'The nobility of sight' (1954). Philosophy's obsession with 'clarity', with representations, and the fundamental assumption that philosophy's task is 'to hold, as 'twere, the mirror up to nature' in the words of Hamlet, all rely on a form of visual bias at the very heart of philosophical inquiry, something Richard Rorty expounds in his *Philosophy and the Mirror of Nature* (1979). Another essay by Jay, 'Scopic regimes of modernity', furthers these ideas about the power of the pictorial and 'the ubiquity of vision as the master sense of the modern era' (1988: 3) through rich examples from art history. One danger of such narratives is that they revaluate non-visual sensory regimes and simplistically counterpose them to vision, or elevate them beyond sight. For example, at one stage Jay suggests that touch offers an alternative model against the ubiquity of vision:

> [T]ouch allows a more benign interaction. Instead of the distance between subject and object congenial to sight, touch restores the proximity of self and other, who then is understood as neighbor. It also entails a more intimate relation to the world. (1994: 517)

Counterposing touch with vision, hands with eyes in this way is a rather unhelpful opposition, and reappraising touch as automatically more proximate and intimate is problematic (examined further in Paterson 2007). Nevertheless, with Rorty, Jay, and others recognising and problematising the centrality of vision for philosophy and culture, the emphasis remains on what is represented to the eye and the visual imagination, which stands in an uneasy relationship with the absence of the visual or the dysfunction of the eye. The place of blindness in philosophy and culture, in other words, remains peripheral, marginalised.

Dioptrique and the blind man's stick

In many ways it all starts with René Descartes, and the origins of a distinct theory of visual perception. While he had most probably been working on his text *Dioptrique* (translated variously as 'Optics', 'Dioptrics', or 'On optics'; see McDonough 2016) from around 1620, and circulated it in draft form to philosophers and natural scientists, it was finally published in France alongside other essays on meteorology and geometry as part of the famous *Discourse on Method* in 1637. *Dioptrique* is an extremely impressive work in its own right. It consists of ten 'discourses' that explain variously the laws of optics, the properties of light, and optical phenomena. Indeed, much of this work was original and contributed the first credible scientific explanation of rainbows, as well as introducing the new study of analytic geometry. It offered the first printed mathematical description of the law of refraction, although the phenomenon had independently been discovered by an English astronomer in 1601 and a Dutch mathematician in 1621, according to Grayling's biography of Descartes (2005: 106–7). The third discourse deals directly with the mechanisms of human vision. It must be remembered that explanations for visual perception until then remained indebted to earlier Scholastic Aristotelianism, which mixed Christian theology with classical philosophy from late antiquity, and they were starting to make sense of theories of medicine and optics from the Middle East, including Al-Kindi and the experiments of Alhazen (see e.g. Lindberg 1976). It is against this background that Descartes' mechanistic ambition stands out. He proposes an anatomical description of the various parts of the eye, including the pupil, the interior 'humours', and the optic nerve. In the fourth discourse Descartes provides an account of the senses in general, explaining 'how the mind, located in the brain, can thus receive impressions of external objects through the mediation of the nerves' (1965: 87). The fifth discourse explains how light enters through the pupil of the eye and is refracted by the interior humours to form an inverted image at the back of the eye, on the retina. The sixth discourse attempts to identify how objects of sight are apprehended, offers an explanation for the visual perception of distance, and demonstrates how human vision is prone to error.

This synopsis is provided for three reasons. First, Descartes' attempt to offer explanations for the mechanisms of optics encompasses the physics of light and refraction, yet places the eye, the retina, and the nerves all within an ambitiously overarching mechanistic philosophy. The subject matter of *Dioptrique* overlapped with Descartes' more foundational project, *Traité du monde et de la lumière* ['The world or treatise on light'], which offered no less than 'a general mechanistic account of the universe including the formation, transmission, and reception of light' (McDonough 2016). He was forced to abandon *The World* in 1633 because Galileo's work on heliocentric motion and mechanics had led to his imprisonment by the Church, but Descartes published material from the project in other forms, including *Dioptrique* and the *Discourse on Method* in 1637. Secondly, Descartes' work on optics is to be considered alongside his other works on natural science, as they each show a critical awareness of the scientific method. This awareness would find its fullest realisation in the *Discourse on Method*, the full title of which concerns 'the method for rightly directing one's reason and searching for truth in the sciences' (1965: 3). Therefore, mechanisms of light and optics might be considered indissociable from his reflexive inquiry into truth, method, and certainty. Thirdly, Descartes the man, and the Cartesian dualism between mind and body for which he is justly famous, are too often reduced to caricature. In undergraduate classes around the world, in disciplines as diverse as cultural studies or the social sciences, Descartes assumes the role of a straw man against whom more fashionable theories are contrasted and counterposed. Nonetheless, the understanding that vision is as much to do with the brain and the nerves as with the eye shows how impressively modern Descartes' overarching project was, tying in mechanisms of optics with mechanisms of the human eye and of mind. His *L'Homme* ['Treatise of man'], written in 1633 and intended to be published in *The World*, pushed out the limits of mechanism by suggesting that all of God's creation, including that most accomplished creation, human beings, was equally reducible to the interactions between mechanisms. With Galileo imprisoned for heresy, the *Treatise of Man* could only be published posthumously in 1664.

With Descartes' emphasis on mechanisms of light and optics, and the functioning of the mind and the body, what place is there for dysfunction of the eye mechanisms, for the loss of vision, for blindness? At one point in the sixth discourse of *Dioptrique*, in a passage addressing errors in perception and visual hallucinations, the start of his explanation is remarkably prescient: 'it is the mind which sees, not the eye; and it can see immediately only through the intervention of the brain' (1965: 108). A more pithy explanation of the difference between sight and vision, where sight is a result of optic mechanisms including the lens and patterns of light on the retina, and vision involves the brain in a larger perceptual and processing system dealing with the sensory data that comes through the eye, would not be realised for some considerable time.

Descartes does consider blindness, in passing, in the first discourse of *Dioptrique*. However, this is not to counterpose blindness against vision, or even to consider blindness in terms of eye function or dysfunction. First, he asks sighted readers to place themselves in the position of being in a dark and unfamiliar place, late at night, where a stick might be used as an aid. He then invokes the hypothetical man born blind as an example of someone who habitually uses a stick as an extension of his senses:

> It has sometimes doubtless happened to you, while walking in the night without a light through places which are a little difficult, that it became necessary to use a stick in order to guide yourself; and you may then have been able to notice that you felt, through the medium of this stick, the diverse objects placed around you, and that you could even tell whether there were trees, or stones, or sand, or water, or grass, or mud, or any other such thing. True, this kind of sensation is somewhat confused and obscure in those who do not have long practice with it; but consider it in those born blind, who have made use of it all their lives: with them, you will find it is so perfect and so

exact, that one might almost say that they see with their hands, or that their stick is the organ of some sixth sense given to them in place of sight. (Descartes 1965: 67)

Much of the language in this first discourse is flavoured with tactility, and the use of sticks. However, this is rather misleading and some contextual analysis is necessary. In this passage Descartes refers to a form of tactile perception that is 'confused and obscure' to those sighted subjects who are unused to discerning their environment through touch, and this has a famous counterpoint in the *Meditations on First Philosophy* of 1644, where at various points he states that our epistemic certainty is initially grounded in 'clear and distinct perception'. But as the *Meditations* proceed, certainty about what appears to the senses as clear and distinct, and therefore intuitive or self-evident, becomes corroded. Previously an Aristotelian 'sense-based epistemology', as Hatfield (1986: 46) puts it, had taken root in Scholastic philosophy, distilled in the Peripatetic axiom 'There is nothing in the intellect that was not first in the senses', and elaborated upon by St Thomas Aquinas in his *Quaestiones disputatae de veritate* ['Disputed questions on truth', 2.13.9], written between 1256 and 1259. This epistemological legacy is what Descartes ends up reversing completely as the *Meditations* continues, and consequently the senses 'are demoted from chief stewards of knowledge' to 'a more mundane, pragmatic function as navigational guides and arbiters of bodily benefits and harms' (Hatfield 1986: 56). Descartes' awareness of illusions, and the occasions on which he has been deceived by his senses, lead him to reverse the Peripatetic axiom, and to consider innate ideas ('the intellect') as prior to error-prone sensations.

Given the context of his suspicion regarding the senses and the sense organs, and his interest in mechanistic explanations as the foundation of natural science, it should be evident that Descartes' concern in *Dioptrique* is decidedly peripheral to any nameless blind figure who feels their way through unfamiliar grounds. In considering the blind as those who 'see with their hands', as Judovitz explains, 'Descartes equates vision with touch, a sense which he considers to be more certain and less vulnerable to error than vision' (1993: 71). Sight may still be the noblest of the senses but, in the pursuit of epistemological certainty, touch is a more dependable model. Descartes placed his example in the first discourse specifically to illustrate a physical model of the behaviour of light as it travels through the eye and stimulates the nerves. He asks the reader to consider the passage of light into the eye as nothing other than 'a certain movement or action, very rapid and very lively, which passes toward our eyes through the medium of the air [...] in the same manner that the movement or resistance of the bodies that this blind man encounters is transmitted to his hand through the medium of his stick' (1965: 67). Part of this explanation is to advance the notion, novel at the time, that the passage of light was instantaneous, travelling through air and transparent bodies in a linear manner, like a stick striking perpendicularly to the ground, affirming the ground's continual presence and immediacy. But the main purpose is to reveal, by analogy with touch, the visual process as pure, one might say 'blind', mechanism. As Judovitz puts it: 'By taking recourse to blindness and the "seeing stick", Descartes transforms seeing into a purely mechanical operation, one determined by the position and activity of the seeing subject in regard to the passive object of sight' (1993: 71).

Descartes' primary concern, then, is not the perceived object as such, nor the subject of vision who is inevitably prone to illusion or error. It is the mechanisms of vision, what causes us to see. We might notice in this situation that 'you felt, through the medium of the stick, the diverse objects placed around you, and that you were even able to tell whether they were trees, or stones, or sand, or water, or grass, or mud, or any such thing' (1965: 67). At first, the differentiation and recognition of textures both underfoot and at arm's length would be unfamiliar and non-habitual, and so might seem 'confused and obscure'. But through habit and practice, feeling the world through the hands, feet, and prostheses such as canes can become more discriminating and precise, and provide more refined sensations. Yet in the first and later discourses, Descartes provides explanations for optical phenomena in haptic terms. If the way that light travels through our eyes is likened to the way that a hypothetical blind man touches the objects around him with a cane, this is a model of the way that images are formed in the brain in terms of tactile transmission. Using an elementary theory of the nervous system that finds fuller explanation in his *Treatise of Man* (1664), in the fourth discourse of *Dioptrique* Descartes attempts an explanation for being able to sense the full range of the qualities and attributes of an object. If we have an 'image' of an object in our brain, he says, not only do we assume that the image resembles the actual object perceived in the world, but there are also other associated qualities in the image. Using a well-worn example, we compensate for perspective by not seeing the drawing of a circle presented to us at an angle as an oval. The multitude of qualities that form the 'image' in our brain are explained therefore in terms of a mechanism of direct transmission from sense organs through the nerves to the brain:

> [J]ust as when the blind man [...] touches some object with his cane, it is certain that these objects do not transmit anything to him except that, by making his cane move in different ways according to their different inherent qualities, they likewise and in the same way move the nerves of his hand, and then the places in his brain where these nerves originate [for Descartes, controversially, the pineal gland]. Thus his mind is caused to perceive as many different qualities in these bodies, as there are varieties in the movements that they cause in his brain. (Descartes 1965: 90)

According to this non-visual explanation for the process of vision, one would think that the single-point touch of a stick would limit the analogy. Interestingly, Descartes offers a richness of perception here based on the variation of movements of the stick, contacting different objects at various angles, and presumably receiving varying levels of resistance due to texture. This is plausibly the case for those blind and vision-impaired users of canes who constantly tap the street in front of them. Furthermore, as an explanation for the visual process as a whole, it indicates how the sense organs (eyes, or in this case hands) themselves are only one component. A theory of nervous transmission is being advanced that involves the inclusion of other organs and components in the service of a bodily mechanism. For example, in the opening paragraph of the seventh discourse, Descartes notes that the quality of human vision depends on three 'principles', namely visible objects, external organs, including all bodies 'that we can place between the eye and object', and interior organs such as the brain and nerves (1965: 114). On the way to this, in the third discourse Descartes offers an anatomical description of the parts of the eye, including the pupil, its interior 'humours', and the optic nerve. In the fourth discourse he provides an account of the senses in general, explaining 'how the mind, located in the brain' comes to receive 'impressions of external objects through the mediation of the nerves' (1965: 87). Of course, this explanation is most amenable to the form of transmission through the nerves that occurs through a stick, as noted above. The fifth discourse explores the physics of light entering through the pupil and how it is refracted by the interior humours, forming an inverted image on the retina at the back of the eye. Similarly, in the sixth discourse Descartes' explanation for the way that we automatically 'see' images the right way up, despite their inverse projection, is compared to the way that a hypothetical blind man is able to determine the position of objects at the end of two crossing sticks, despite the position of the hands being differently oriented. In other words, the resistance of a stick striking an object, when felt through the hands, will be interpreted correctly whether there is one stick, two sticks, or two crossing sticks encountering an object. Our brains become habituated so that the resulting image is orientated correctly. Descartes explains this is through an apparently commonsensical approach whereby the nerves in the hand touching the stick 'cause a certain change' in the blind man's brain (1965: 104) so that the mind 'can turn its attention to' the objects that are touched by the stick, and feel them rather than the already known location of his two hands (1965: 105). Thus we feel the strike of a lamppost or a pillarbox through the cane, for example, and become immediately aware of them as perceived objects rather than as a series of localised sensations in the hands. Our minds become extended through the sticks.

Again, these insights concerning tactility and its extension are then brought to bear on visual perception, as the directly felt yet mediated nature of the experience of touching with a stick is likened by Descartes to the way that we filter out our head and eye movements in the visual perception of an object. Returning to the analogy of two crossed sticks, he directly compares this to having two eyes: 'And just as this blind man does not judge that a body is double, although he touches it with his two hands, so likewise when both our eyes are disposed in the manner which is required in order to carry our attention toward one and the same location, they need only cause us to see a single object there, even though a picture of it is formed in each of our eyes' (1965: 105). The experience of seeing something is felt as direct and unmediated, yet in both touch and vision, as perceivers, we are unaware of any actual bodily mediations. Later, in the twentieth century, philosophers would return to the figure of the blind man with a cane. A noted passage in Maurice Merleau-Ponty's *Phenomenology of Perception* revisits how external objects such the blind man's cane become an habitual extension of their body, and thereby become literally 'incorporated' (1992: 166). It could be said that he re-reverses the Peripatetic axiom, using a familiar analogy in order to argue vociferously, against Descartes, for a more embodied form of consciousness.

As we have seen, Descartes' explanations of purely optical phenomena are cast in tactile terms for a reason. For the reader to be convinced, however, the analogy presupposes some form of translatability, if not actual equivalence, between the senses, so that it is entirely conceivable that transfer from one 'sense' or sensory modality (e.g. vision) to another (e.g. touch) is possible. Writing as he was half a century prior to the formulation of Molyneux's question, we appreciate that Descartes is neither interested in the senses as a path to knowledge, nor in hypothetical questions of transfer between the tactile and visual data of sensation, labelled 'cross-modal' perception in the psychology literature (e.g. Gregory and Wallace 1963: 37; Gregory 2004: 836). But Descartes' explanatory mechanism does rely on exploiting the potential for the recognition of reconciling the different realms of sensory experience, according to touch and to vision, for the reader at least. Descartes' sensory analogy of a tactile form of vision, a 'seeing stick', therefore to some extent still relies upon the recognition of a pre-existing ability to substitute one sense for another, what neuroscientist Bach-y-Rita terms 'sensory substitution' (Bach-y-Rita et al. 1969). This is especially the case for blindness or deafness, where there is an absent or heavily impaired sense, and where rehabilitation technologies like those pioneered by Bach-y-Rita can substitute for that missing sense. Descartes' sensory analogy, although uninterested in the sensory phenomena themselves, still manages to engage the hypothetical curiosity of the reader and open a path of inquiry ahead of the Molyneux question. Albeit in the service of explaining the mechanisms of optics and the pathways of light through the eye and into the brain, his analogy may still prompt us to question whether we have distinct, independently working senses, where some form of cross-modal transfer is possible. Or, conversely, whether the nature of perception is essentially amodal, entailing that sensory information is prior to, or independent of, any particular sense modality, in line with some classical models of sense perception. Variants of these questions will form the basis for thought experiments, and for other hypothetical blind men, as the next chapters unfold.

If Descartes' analogy of 'seeing with the hands' is only incidentally interested in blindness per se, a philosophical concern with actual blindness and the experience of being blind will not occur until over a hundred years later, in Denis Diderot's *Lettre sur les aveugles* of 1749. Diderot refers to Descartes' same analogy concerning hands and eyes and develops the idea of 'seeing with sticks' (1916a: 74) in a different direction, as we shall see. But instead of the hypothetical blind man of *Dioptrique*, the blind man who Diderot goes to interview in the small town of Puiseaux is asked directly how he conceives of the function and purpose of eyes. The *Lettre* somewhat validates Descartes' interpretation of touch in terms of vision, and certainly the tactile model of vision comes through in some of the blind subject's answers to Diderot. While Descartes' explanatory model in no way equates with actual experiences of blindness, Diderot's focus throughout the *Lettre* is exactly on those experiences. Noticing Descartes' use of tactile imagery to explain optical phenomena, then, Diderot chastises him for his misunderstanding of blindness:

> Madame, only turn to Descartes' *Dioptrics*, and there you will see the phenomena of sight illustrated by those of touch, and the plates full of men busied in seeing with sticks. Descartes, and all the later writers, have not been able to give us clearer ideas of vision; and that great philosopher was, in this respect, no more superior to the blind man than a common man who has the use of his eyes. (Diderot 1916a: 73)

It is all very well admonishing other philosophers for not understanding blindness. But Diderot artfully develops the 'seeing with sticks' analogy to equate the touch-space of the stick around the body to something like a visual field. For example, through his purported interviews with a range of actual, and not hypothetical, blind figures in the *Lettre*, he finds that the well-known phenomenon of occlusion, where an object's appearance is hidden or altered by another closer object in the line of sight, is also present in touch. This is revealed by the blind man from Puiseaux in response to one of Diderot's questions: 'When I place my hand between your eyes and an object, my hand is present to you but the object is absent. The same thing happens when I reach for one thing with my stick and come across another' (1916a: 73). Diderot has much more to say about experiences of blindness, and chapter 5 explores how his project lies between philosophical and psychological inquiry.

Close vision with the fingertips

Descartes was aware of the cornea, the retina, and the functioning of the lens. Kepler had proved in *Ad vitellionem paralipomena* (1604) that the lens produced an inverted image on the back of the retina. In the fifth discourse of *Dioptrique*, entitled 'Of the images that form on the back of the eye', Descartes advocated seeing this for ourselves by 'taking the eye from a recently deceased man, or for want of that, of an ox or some other large animal' (1985: 91), removing the back of the eye, and letting light pass through on to an eggshell or piece of paper. There we would see, 'not perhaps without admiration and pleasure' (1985: 93), an inverted and perspectively correct image whose size can be altered by squeezing the eye. The mechanics of optics laid bare, made manifest through a material and meaty instantiation. But further anatomical components of the eye and their specific functions would be discovered subsequently that are also potentially relevant to a Cartesian tactile model of vision. For example, the macula is an ovoid area near the centre of the retina that affords greater visual acuity. Within the macula itself is a small indentation in the eyeball, the fovea (from Latin, 'small pit') which contains the largest concentration of cone cells for colour vision and is responsible for the high-resolution vision known as central vision necessary for reading, sewing, or other close vision tasks. To pursue further the analogy between hands and eyes, therefore, it has been argued that this acute vision, or foveation, has some equivalence with the more fine-grained tactile acuity of the fingertips. This heightened tactile acuity was noticed by Diderot. If foveation or the equivalent of central vision occurs within the fingertips, the hand and its prostheses (say, a blind man's stick or cane) imply more peripheral and indistinct vision. In the *Lettre*, Diderot does acknowledge something like a precursor to this foveation analogy:

> If ever a philosopher, blind and deaf from his birth, were to construct a man after the fashion of Descartes, I can assure you, madam, that he would put the seat of the soul at the fingers' ends, for thence the greater part of the sensations and all his knowledge are derived. (1916a: 87)

For, although touch is distributed throughout the body, and the skin is the largest sense organ, the more accurate and discriminating aspect of our touch perception comes from the hands, and especially the fingertips, due to the increased density of nerve endings. In medical science, this was confirmed by surgeon and anatomist Charles Sherrington in 1906 (see Wilson 1999: 97). The extension of the analogy to fingertips becomes highly significant in sensory substitution, particularly in the case of Braille and later sensory substitution devices. It seems only natural to expect an analogy between the increased visual resolution of the macula and the heightened tactile resolution of the hands, say, and correspondingly between the high-definition optical discrepancy of the fovea and the highly discriminatory tactile sensing of the fingertips.

In reconsidering vision through the analogy with touch, or what Appelbaum thinks of as purposefully donning 'the cloak of blindness' (1995: 13), Descartes in turn sought to unveil the mechanisms underlying vision that foregrounded the role of the brain, and an elementary concept of a nervous system, instead of solely optical processes. The cloak, or the guise of a blind man with a stick, is only ever an explanatory tactic. However unwittingly, along the way *Dioptrique* opens up a pathway to think about sensory substitution in functional terms, that is, achieving a functional equivalent for the eye through the hands, the cane, and later Braille. A stronger and more fully realised version of the argument for sensory substitution would be articulated just fifty years later through Molyneux. The debate that Molyneux initiated would take Descartes' idea of the mind being the perceiving entity, as opposed to the sense organs, further, while switching back the polarity of the Peripatetic axiom regarding the significance of the senses versus the intellect, of experience rather than rationality, to its original formulation. This process occurred for a while, at least, as a wave of British empiricism took off through Locke and his anti-Cartesian advocates in France.

As we have seen, rather than an analogue that assumes some form of equivalence between the senses, the idea of an exact interchangeability between the senses negates the particularities of each sense modality. This is an invitation that Berkeley would take up in the course of his answer to Locke and Molyneux's question in 1709, the focus of the following chapter. The mechanisms that comprise the eye, including the lens, cornea, and humours, are inessential in themselves and could be replaced by alternatives, for sight is a product of mind, a matter of conceptual processing, and consequently one stream of information can replace another without loss. Appelbaum summarises the implication for that schema: 'One kind of sensory input may be used in place of another – sound, taste, or touch can be used in place of sight. None presents the different; all present the same. Perfect interchangeability holds among the senses' (1995: 25). Not surprising perhaps, given Berkeley's idealism, that blindness would be downplayed, rendered less significant, since the same information could be obtained without sight through other means. Apart from the augmentation of vision through spectacles in Berkeley's time, this interchangeability would have been largely a hypothetical consideration, but recent decades have introduced technologies such as retinal prostheses that significantly alter and re-route the optical processes of the eye by direct stimulation of the optic nerve in order to produce vision. The idea of perfect interchangeability might be the logical progression of a Cartesianism that posits mind as the thing that sees, but it is not at all what Descartes argues.

Chapter 2

'Suppose a man born blind...': Cubes and Spheres, Hands and Eyes

The unanswered question

Decades after Descartes' philosophical speculations about blindness in *Dioptrique*, a resurgence of interest in blindness occurred across the channel in England, sparking a series of celebrated debates and dialogues between intellectuals in Britain and France that included such figures as Berkeley (1709), Hutcheson (1728), Bouillier (1737), Jurin (1738), La Mettrie (1745), Condillac (1746), Diderot (1749), Reid (1764), and Leibniz (1765). What became known in the philosophy literature as either 'Molyneux's question' or the 'Molyneux problem' was regarded by the influential historian of philosophy Ernst Cassirer in 1951 as the central question of eighteenth-century epistemology and psychology (in Gallagher 2005: 153). This chapter provides more historical focus on the question and its implications, the better to justify Cassirer's claim. Of course, while Molyneux's seemingly naive and straightforward philosophical question initially concerns blindness, the question is asked hypothetically, between a philosopher and a scientist, in order to clarify the relationship between perception through the senses and the certainty of knowledge concerning objects in the world. This chapter opens with Molyneux's initial concern of his hypothetical blind man, and pursues its philosophical ramifications within the immediate context of debates between the rationalism of Descartes' method, which looked to place reason at the heart of the philosophical and scientific enterprise, and the empiricism of his British philosophical counterparts Locke and Berkeley, who argued against the existence of any pre-existing or innate knowledge in order to see how more complex ideas and concepts can arise from simple experiences. For, prior to any recorded cataract operations or opthalmic interventions, and prior to any formation of a properly experimental psychology, this question and its immediate aftermath initiated, as we saw, a 'proto-psychology' in Grosrichard's (2012) words, but also sets up the philosophical framework in subsequent chapters that examine, first, the empirical and scientifically verifiable treatments of blind subjects after Cheselden's surgery in 1728, and secondly, the ensuing cross-channel epistemological debate involving Diderot, Voltaire, and others based on this and other evidence.

Although his original question in the form of a letter to John Locke in 1688 was ignored, in 1692 the Irishman William Molyneux posed the question to Locke for a second time, following the publication and success of the first edition of Locke's celebrated *An Essay Concerning Human Understanding* in 1690. To remind ourselves, in Riskin's pithy version the question asks: 'If a man, blind from birth, suddenly gained vision, could he tell a sphere from a cube by sight alone on the basis of a lifetime of solely tactile experience?' (2002: 23). In *Dioptrique*, as we saw, Descartes had hypothesised that the blind 'see with their hands' to justify a mechanistic model of vision. But how the congenitally blind, those without any prior visual experience, perceive space and perform the transfer of tactile to visual information, or conceive of vision and the function of the eye, remains central to the Molyneux question. My concern here is not simply to recapitulate previous discussions of the Molyneux question in philosophy (e.g. Morgan 1977; Degenaar 1996) or in experimental psychology (e.g. von Senden 1960; Jones 1975). In the debate between its early interlocutors Locke, Molyneux, and Berkeley, the initial answers to Molyneux's question suggest potentially differing viewpoints on these issues, and subsequent contributions in their wake have attempted to resolve them definitively. But within its immediate historical context the Molyneux problem cuts to the heart of Locke's philosophy of mind, directly prompting Berkeley to write *An Essay Towards a New Theory of Vision* (1709) in response, as they begin to unravel the complexity of those processes underlying perception, and how complex judgements and concepts can be formed from simple sensations or ideas within everyday experience. With Molyneux as the initial catalyst, and during a period with no shortage of treatises on optics, Locke instigated a novel direction of inquiry into vision and its relationship to the other sense modalities, leading him to be esteemed the 'Father of English Psychology' three centuries after his birth (e.g. Edgell 1932: 169). The significance of the Molyneux question for our larger unfolding narrative since Descartes of the spatial imaginary of the blind by the sighted, or what the blind 'see', cannot be understated. Presently we examine the philosophical root of the issue and see why, as Josipovici observes, in thinking about blindness after Molyneux 'we are all heirs of the seventeenth century' (1996: 69).

This chapter considers how a series of mostly British philosophers after Molyneux, including Locke, Synge, Berkeley, and Reid, placed great emphasis on the possibility of translatability between sensory modalities in order to develop increasingly sophisticated models of perception and its role in knowledge acquisition. The unfolding dialogue is mostly summarised in this chapter in chronological terms from Molyneux's question onwards, centring on the relationship between vision and touch in knowledge acquisition for hypothetical blind subjects. In the decades following Molyneux's question, attempts to answer it slowly coagulated around certain key philosophical positions: first, whether there are underlying universal concepts dissociated from any particular sense modality, yet which are equally available to consciousness whether the subject is blind, deaf, or whatever; and secondly, whether the particularity of the knowledge available to each sense modality is at least partially translatable to other modalities. Note that the first does not necessarily preclude the second. Much of the epistemological inquiry after Molyneux assumes the generation of more complex and abstract ideas from a subject's exposure to simple sensations, but also that, through repeated exposure to such sensations, cross-modal perceptions permit subjects to recognise the objects of touch through the mechanisms of sight, for example.

Locke's dark room

After his initial query in 1688, Molyneux's question was posed again in slightly altered form in 1692, and this version is what Locke quoted and responded to in Book II, Chapter IX of the second edition of the *Essay* entitled 'Of perception'. Locke saw how the question and its answer might advance his argument about the role of experience in perceiving objects in the external world. Looking at a round object, say, how do we judge it as flat or three-dimensional, concave or convex? Locke was interested in the role that experience of raw sensations played in forming perceptions and concepts of the world, or 'ideas' in Locke's terminology. 'Ideas' in this sense resemble our modern usage of the word, but have a somewhat convoluted heritage. Locke's contemporary Malebranche, as Descartes before him, was dealing with the legacy of medieval thought on such matters, considering the nature of ideas as mind–body interactions whose original cause or progenitor was God, a philosophy known as Occasionalism, first articulated by St Thomas Aquinas in the thirteenth century and revisited by Malebranche in the seventeenth. Locke's advocacy of experience and rejection of innatism required that ideas originate not directly from God but from our own immediate sensory experience. Neither is this an original formulation, for Locke's declaration that 'perception is the first operation of all our intellectual faculties, and the inlet of all knowledge in our minds' (*Essay* II.IX.15) echoes the Peripatetic axiom of Aquinas, 'There is nothing in the intellect that was not first in the senses.' Whereas for Aquinas information from the senses allows us to deduce abstract universal principles through the action of the intellect, for Locke sensations are the starting point for a process of induction, are not God-given, and so have their own existence. Ideas are 'whatsoever is the object of the understanding when a man thinks' (*Essay* I.I.8), and the mind 'hath no other immediate object but its own *ideas*' (*Essay* IV.I.1, original emphasis), says Locke. Thus ideas are not simply raw or unprocessed sensations but have object-like properties, an existence that the mind fixes or determines (for more on this see Yolton 1984: 88ff.).

From Locke's perspective we might ask how patches and patterns of light, shadow, and colour perceived through the eyes become routinely and unreflectingly interpreted as seemingly material objects with physical, material properties perceivable through touch, like weight and hardness. How is this achieved without the need to grasp or manipulate for verification? What separates our visual apprehension of a two-dimensional painting or photograph of an apple, say, with its colours, shapes, and shades, from the directly perceived actual apple standing before us? For 'the *ideas we receive by sensation are often* in grown people *altered by the judgment*, without our taking notice of it', says Locke (*Essay* II.IX.8, original emphasis). Through what he terms 'habitual custom', exposure to repeated associations between the three-dimensional material properties of objects and the two-dimensional light patterns that enter the eyes alters the way we see and interact with them. In Book II of the *Essay* Locke professed that at birth our mind has no innate ideas, famously likening it to a blank slate or 'white paper' (II.I.2), following in a tradition since Aristotle and Aquinas of considering the brain as devoid of innate ideas or rules at birth. If simple ideas are gained from sensation, complex ideas are formed from them by processes of combination, division, generalisation, and abstraction. Such was the radical cornerstone of Lockean empiricism, a concentration on the role of sensory experience in philosophy that was contrary to the rationalism of Descartes or Leibniz, where intellectual certainty was gained not through the senses but through the forms of deductive reasoning pursued in mathematics and geometry, for example. Locke is interested in the role of experience in unconsciously shaping our present perception of objects, and makes references to memory (in *Essay*, Chapter X), and to associations between the senses in the perception of objects. Conventionally enough, Locke's examples are predominantly visual throughout the *Essay*, and Yolton notices how Locke's writing 'often uses visual and even optical language to describe perception' (1984: 125). For example, and consistent with Descartes, sight is 'the most comprehensive of all our senses, conveying to our minds the *ideas* of light and colours, which are peculiar only to that sense' (*Essay* II.IX.9, original emphasis). Locke's emphasis on visual language and examples extends from the more conventional metaphor of the blank slate to a more fleshed-out, three-dimensional model for thinking about the role of the senses in the production of knowledge in the mind. This was Locke's example of the 'dark room', the literal translation of *camera obscura* in Latin, a space closed off from any surrounding light. As a visual metaphor that counterposes the darkness of unknowing with the light of ideas, the intromission of light into a dark, empty receptacle is consistent with standard Enlightenment tropes.

The usually room-sized camera obscura, a precursor to the photographic camera, had one small opening that allowed light from the outside to project an inverted image of the outside world on to the two-dimensional surface of a floor or the opposite wall. It became historically established as a model of the optics of vision when Robert Hooke wrote his *Lectures on Light* in 1680, and Hooke discusses how previously Della Porta, Kepler, and Descartes in *Dioptrique* each employed this model to explain the workings of the eye (see Lindberg 1976; Crary 1990; 1999). However, this phenomenon of optical projection was discussed much earlier by scientists and philosophers such as Euclid, Aristotle, Alhazen, and Bacon. Variants of the apparatus were also used for the purpose of generating realistic linear perspective within artistic practice, beginning with the architectural drawings of Brunelleschi in the fifteenth century, and later in the paintings of Vermeer and Canaletto. For this reason, Hooke also referred to the camera as a 'perspective box' (in Yolton 1984: 125), as if what was projected into the room was an incontrovertibly objective representation of the outside world. Molyneux in his *Dioptrica nova* (1692) associated it not with artistic use, however, but with the shallow entertainments of the peepshow and the magic lantern (Crary 1990: 33 n. 10). A more serious scientific use occurred in one of Newton's experiments in *Opticks*, when a glass prism was placed within the aperture of 'a very dark Chamber' so that 'a colour'd image of the Sun' (1730: 21–2) formed on its opposite wall. As a result of contemporaneous developments in anatomical and physiological knowledge, then, the camera obscura worked not only as a commonplace analogy for the optical mechanism of the human eye but, especially in Newton's *Opticks* and Locke's *Essay*, also as an 'interiorized and disembodied subject' (Crary 1990: 40). In other words, the projection of an inverted image on to a two-dimensional surface modelled the observation of empirical phenomena, but simultaneously reflected back to the observer their detachment from the process of seeing, their 'reflective introspection and self-observation' (Crary 1990: 40). In such a way, the process of understanding what we see is at one remove, likened by Locke to 'the face at the perspective box scanning the images on the wall of the box' (Yolton 1984: 126).

So for Locke the camera obscura has already shifted from modelling the optical processes involved when light enters the eye through the lens and inversely projects on to the retina. Instead, it becomes an instantiation of the epistemological relationship between sensory experiences (not just vision) and the faculty of 'understanding', knowledge of concepts from the outside world, or what we now term 'cognition':

> I pretend not to teach, but to inquire; and therefore cannot but confess here again that external and internal sensation are the only passages I can find of knowledge to the understanding. These alone, as far as I can discover, are the windows by which light is let into this *dark room*. For, methinks, the *understanding* is not much unlike a closet wholly shut from light, with only some little openings left, to let in external visible resemblances, or *ideas* of things without: which, would they but stay there, and lie so orderly as to be found upon occasion, it would very much resemble the understanding of a man, in reference to all objects of sight, and the *ideas* of them. (*Essay* II.XI.17, original emphasis)

Locke's notion that the human understanding forms complex ideas from simple sensations in this passage is likened in strongly visual terms to the familiar form of the dark closet or chamber with only pinholes and door cracks to admit light. In turn, this involves our perceptions of objects via the various bodily senses at our disposal, notwithstanding any sensory loss or impairment within an individual.

The inherent empiricist assumptions behind this analogy are established by virtue of the room being initially completely dark, indicating the absence of innate ideas or pre-existing principles. Accordingly, experiences and combinatory sensations from outside the room are necessitated to form ideas *ab initio*.

Indeed, prior to the introduction of the Molyneux question in the *Essay*, Locke looks briefly to another example of blindness and restored sight to further cement his opposition to innate ideas, claiming that there is nothing in the mind apart from present 'ideas' (his terminology for perceptions, or objects of the understanding) or the memory of past 'ideas'. There remains no vestige of anything innate. Uncompromisingly he asserts: 'For what is not either actually in view, or in the memory, is in the mind no way at all, and is all one as if it had never been there' (*Essay* I.IV.20). Locke offers an illustration by way of the visual memory of colour, and anticipates the surgical procedure known as 'couching', the removal of a cataract by downward displacement of the lens of the eye. Locke considers the hypothetical case of a child who has functioning colour vision who then develops cataracts, or as he puts it, 'then cataracts shut the windows, and he is forty or fifty years perfectly in the dark' (*Essay* I.IV.20). His choice of similes is noteworthy, equating windows with eyes that let in light or, if dysfunctional, produce darkness. During this extended period of hypothetical blindness the child has no experience of colour, and its memory of colour steadily degrades, then becomes lost. Locke proffers the fruits of his own discussion with a supposedly actual, existing blind subject to advance the argument further against innate ideas:

> This was the case of a blind man I once talked with, who lost his sight by the small-pox, when he was a child, and had no more notion of colours, than one born blind. I ask, whether any one can say this man had then any ideas of colours in his mind, any more than one born blind? and, I think, nobody will say, that either of them had in his mind any idea of colours at all. His cataracts are couched, and then he has the ideas (which he remembers not) of colours, *de novo*, by his restored sight, conveyed to his mind, and that without any consciousness of a former acquaintance. And these now he can revive, and call to mind in the dark. (*Essay* I.IV.20)

The implication is that visual memories fade, become forgotten, even the face of a loved one or a colour in its entirety. After the cataract operation, and exposed once again to visual experience, such visual memories can be remade and persist in the darkness of night or when the eyes are closed. The memory of colour and other visual properties persists because the subject retains the capacity to see those objects of memory in the near future, thereby continuing to forge associations (what Locke termed 'habitual customs' of perception), according with his epistemological model of the dark room of the understanding.

Molyneux's question and Locke's answer

William Molyneux was born in Dublin and trained for three years in London as a lawyer, but in an era of great advances in the physics and technologies of optics his interests were swept up in philosophy, optics, and astronomy. He was the translator into English of Descartes' *Six Metaphysical Meditations, Wherein it is Proved that there is a God* in 1680, and in 1683 he founded the Dublin Philosophical Society. Six years before his death he published the first major treatise on optics in English, *Dioptrica nova* (1692). While he is primarily known as a philosophical footnote because of his correspondence with Locke, the *Dioptrica nova* followed Descartes' *Dioptrique* by proposing answers to several questions regarding the mechanisms of sight and refraction of light through lenses, ahead of Newton's *Opticks*. Molyneux's book contributed to this scholarship and 'showed a thorough understanding of the dioptrics of the eye', even proposing 'corrections for myopia and presbyopia' (Wade and Gregory 2006b: 1580). More significantly, Molyneux was 'the cousin and husband of blind women' according to his biographer Simms (in Riskin 2002: 23), and consequently his question to Locke was prompted by his wife's blindness (Wade and Gregory 2006a: 1437). Nevertheless, Molyneux's question concerns the hypothetical case of a man born blind yet who crucially has extensive experience of tactile interactions with objects, and whose vision is restored suddenly through unspecified means at a time before cataract operations could answer this definitively.

Molyneux's letter to Locke of 7 July 1688 was written in response to an abstract of Locke's larger *Essay* published two years earlier in the *Bibliothèque universelle & historique*, an encyclopaedia edited by Jean Le Clerc. The problem is posed initially in the letter in this way:

> A Problem Proposed to the Author of the *Essai Philosophique concernant L'Entendement*
>
> A Man, being born blind, and having a Globe and a Cube, nigh of the same bignes, Committed into his Hands, and being taught or Told, which is Called the Globe, and which the Cube, so as easily to distinguish them by his Touch or Feeling; Then both being taken from Him, and Laid on a Table, Let us Suppose his Sight Restored

to Him; Whether he Could, by his Sight, and before he touch them, know which is the Globe and which the Cube? Or Whether he Could know by his Sight, before he stretch'd out his Hand, whether he Could not Reach them, tho they were Removed 20 or 1000 feet from Him? (Molyneux 1688)

Although initially ignored, the subsequent correspondence between Molyneux and Locke offered the opportunity to restate the question, and for Locke to realise its significance. The altered version published in the second edition of Locke's *Essay* is worded differently and, significantly, removes the last sub-question concerning judgement of distances through vision alone without touch:

> Suppose a man born blind, and now adult, and taught by his touch to distinguish between a cube and a sphere of the same metal, and nighly of the same bigness, so as to tell, when he felt one and the other, which is the cube, which the sphere. Suppose then the cube and sphere placed on a table, and the blind man be made to see: quaere, whether by his sight before he touched them, he could now distinguish and tell which is the globe, which the cube? (*Essay* II.IX.8)

The question was posed decades before Cheselden's first celebrated cataract operation, and any definitive scientific answer would therefore have to wait. Even then, the evidence remained largely inconclusive. But the path for an empirical (that is, experimental) answer to an empiricist problem was paved by Locke, based on his conception of 'ideas'. To varying degrees, Locke and then Berkeley had suggested the role of non-visual experience within visual perception such that we learn to perceive visual space by associating it with other sensations, including touch. This had remained only of theoretical interest until Molyneux 'provided the spur to resolve a question of empiricist philosophy by resort to empirical observations' (Wade and Gregory 2006a: 1438), and led to particular forms of questioning of Cheselden's patient after cataract surgery. Molyneux's question is inevitably couched as a thought experiment, gauging whether the empirical content of tactile experience of the hypothetical blind subject has a specificity of its own, or whether it can be equated a priori with the sensory experience of sight.

The original philosophical debate concerning the origin of ideas and the importance of experience that originally inspired the question, and that was manifest in Locke's analogy of the dark room, altered direction somewhat to 'a new question about sensitive openness to the outside world, even before actual eye surgeries made real the hypothetical blind man given sight' (Riskin 2002: 23). Prior to the surge of cataract operations in the wake of Cheselden, then, a hypothetical answer to the hypothetical question must suffice. Both Molyneux and Locke were in agreement that the answer was negative. Locke paraphrases Molyneux's answer here, before offering his own considered reply:

> For, though he has obtained the experience of how a globe, how a cube affects his touch, yet he has not yet obtained the experience that what affects his touch so or so must affect his sight so or so; or that a protuberant angle in the cube, that pressed his hand unequally, shall appear to his eye as it does in the cube. (*Essay* II.IX.8)

Likewise, Molyneux's answer to his own question is rather concise and clearly extols the necessity of experience in associating the particularity of tactile sensations with those of sight. As we have seen, much of Locke's philosophy in the *Essay* was founded upon the belief that 'ideas' (objects of the understanding) arose from sensations by means of a learned process of 'judgement', so he wastes little time in agreeing with Molyneux:

> I agree with this thinking gentleman, whom I am proud to call my friend, in his answer to this problem; and am of opinion that the blind man, at first sight, would not be able with certainty to say which was the globe, which the cube, whilst he only saw them; though he could unerringly name them by his touch, and certainly distinguish them by the difference of their figures felt. (*Essay* II.IX.8)

He continues, further celebrating our debt to experience within habitual perception, leaving the reader to consider how they 'may be beholden to experience, improvement, and acquired notions' even if we are usually unaware of these factors. Essentially Molyneux had invoked Locke's principle that there is no visual knowledge without visual experience, so the man blind from birth would have no visual 'idea' (in the Lockean sense) of a cube or a sphere. Consequently, according to the Lockean schema, the Molyneux man would simply not have the conceptual resources based on experience to infer from an object affecting his sight that it would affect his sense of touch in any way, and this was because 'the correlation of visual with tactile experiences, and the use of the five senses generally, relied upon a learned process of judgment [in Molyneux's words] "acquired by *Exercise*"' (Riskin 2002: 23).

For the sighted and the newly sighted alike there is a crucial difference between a green disk, a green apple, and a painting of a green apple that strives for a realistic appearance of three-dimensional properties, for example through the representation of shadow and colour gradation according to the position of light sources. In later sections of the *Essay* a learned process of judgement through habitual perception is developed to postulate the habitual concurrence of sensations through different modalities, such as the sound of a gunshot closely succeeding a visual muzzle-flash. In this way, habituation elides the distinctive features of experiences from separate sensory modalities, and does so below the threshold of our conscious awareness. '*Habits*, especially as such are begun very early, come at last to *produce actions in us which often escape our observation*' (*Essay* II.IX.10, original emphasis), Locke says, such that autonomic activities such as blinking, and learned sensory associations such as the muzzle-flash, show in Locke's terms how simple ideas become folded into more complex ideas. Therefore we concentrate less on the immediate ideas or sensations before us, but with increased exposure to learned associations we instantaneously transpose these separate 'ideas' derived from different sensory modalities (the sound, the flash) into our 'judgement' (a gunshot). Or like someone who reads a newspaper or hears a speech, scant notice is taken of the actual characters or sounds, but he concentrates instead upon 'the *ideas* that are excited in him by them':

> This, in many cases by a settled habit, in things whereof we have frequent experience, is performed so constantly and so quick, that we take that for the perception of our sensation which is an *idea* formed by our judgment; so that one, viz. that of sensation, serves only to excite the other, and is scarce taken notice of itself. (*Essay* II.IX.9, original emphasis)

The instantaneity of this process is referred to shortly thereafter with another visual analogy, this time the glance. A demonstration of a complex procedure such as a dance move or mechanical repair shows how this might involve several sensory modalities simultaneously, observed as a series of sensations (ideas) from different modalities, woven almost instantaneously into a comprehensible unity (judgement): 'How, as it were in an instant, do our minds, with one glance, see all the parts of a demonstration, which may very well be called a long one, if we consider the time it will require to put it into words, and step by step show it another?' (*Essay* II.IX.10). In further developing Molyneux's answer Locke later looks to the role of memory, what he terms 'retention', in the ability to recognise the simple ideas from which more complex ideas and judgements are formed, working as the 'storehouse of our *ideas*' (*Essay* II.X.2, original emphasis). But it is the process by which judgement almost instantaneously takes place prior to memory formation or reflection that prompts the question whether the particularity of any sense modality is significant for Locke, or whether it is only the underlying concepts, once intromitted from outside experience like light through the apertures of the camera obscura, built up from 'simple' into more 'complex' ideas, that are of concern. In other words, if Locke's and Molyneux's answer to the Molyneux question is negative, would this not disallow the possibility of what Gregory terms 'cross-modal perception' (Gregory and Wallace 1963), or in the case of sensory impairment, the substitution of one sensory modality for another, Bach-y-Rita's 'sensory substitution' (Bach-y-Rita et al. 1969)?

Locke's negative answer to Molyneux's question has been explained in terms of his overarching argument against innate ideas in principle and, as we have seen, he justified his answer in empirical terms, believing that ideas arose from sensations by means of a learned process of judgement. And we are reminded that sympathetic readers of Locke will agree, in his words, 'how much he may be beholding to experience' (*Essay* II.IX.8) as a result. That ideas arise from combinations of sensations from different sensory modalities, not only vision, has allowed us to consider the mechanisms through which simple visual and non-visual sensations ('ideas') have the potential to form more complex ideas ('judgements' formed through the 'Understanding') in Locke's framework. Given this framework, Locke's answer to the Molyneux question lends itself easily to explanation in terms of the establishment of a correlation ('habitual custom') between non-visual (tactile) and visual sensations for a newly sighted Molyneux man. We now look to Locke's contemporaries and interlocutors for their answers to Molyneux's question, and the changing terms of reference in the subsequent debates until the baton is handed, several decades later, to the French *philosophes*. Nowhere is this more apposite than in the consideration of spatial perception. For what the blind 'see' in visual terms, before or after cataract surgery, is only part of the story. After Locke, the issue becomes more explicitly spatial in Berkeley's attempt to answer Molyneux's question. The manual exploration of successive objects around him that the Molyneux man must perform, along with the ability to navigate through familiar and unfamiliar environments, prompts us to question the role of touch and the non-visual senses in spatial perception.

Responding to Locke and Molyneux: Berkeley and after

Locke's forthrightness and certainty were matched by a certain conceptual innovation in affirming the place of sensory experience in epistemology (the formation of 'ideas') within a larger philosophy of mind ('understanding'). But clearly there would be dissenters and objections to Locke's answer to Molyneux, and some commentators argued for a positive answer, including his contemporary Edward Synge in 1695. Synge proposed his answer directly to Molyneux in a letter that, along with a response from Molyneux, eventually found its way to Locke. Synge's letter appeared in Locke's published correspondence, and his argument is summarised thus:

> The *Image* which upon the first View such a man will frame of a Cube, must needs be this, that it is a body which is not alike in all the parts of its Superficies which consequently must be agreeable to the *idea* which before he had of it and different from that *idea* which he had of a globe. (Locke, *Correspondence* V.496, in Bolton 1994: 79)

Synge's answer depends upon a distinction between 'image' and 'idea', where 'image' is 'that notion only, which a man entertains of a visible thing as it is visible', remaining as patterns of retinal impressions, whereas for Synge the 'idea' follows Locke in being more multifarious, 'every notion of any thing which a man entertains' (in Riskin 2002: 24). According to Synge's answer, the Molyneux subject would have *ideas* in the Lockean sense of cubes and spheres gained through, but not specific to, his sense of touch, and would measure his newly gained images against his old ideas to distinguish cube from sphere. Upon first sight, literally, the once blind man would correlate basic impressions as to visual appearance (images), such as it looks smooth or jagged, has corners or curves, with past sensory experience (ideas) of those objects. Locke replied to Synge's letter with almost artful condescension, writing that their exchange had showed 'how hard it is, for even ingenious men to free themselves from the anticipations of sense' (*Correspondence* V.493, in Bolton 1994: 79). Although easily dismissed by Locke, variations of this argument circulated including one from Leibniz, discussed below. Synge's distinction between visual image and manifold idea, with its reach backward to past sensory experiences, suggests that he is arguing for something akin to the Aristotelian discussions of 'common sensibles'. In *On the Soul* (425a27), for example, common sensibles are objects perceived by several senses at once, but imply a separate faculty that transcends the restrictions of individual sensory modalities, a *sensus communis*, that can form the basis of comparison between sensations and more complex 'ideas' that images are compared to. This 'common sense' has sometimes been conceived as a distinct sense that orders the other senses, an idea revisited in France by Buffon as our 'interior sense' in *Discours sur le nature des animaux* (1753), and by Voltaire in *Dictionnaire philosophique* (1764), and that resurfaces again in various guises in nineteenth- and early twentieth-century medical science (e.g. Wilhelm Wundt's *Gemeinempfindungen* [common sensation], Weber's *Gemeingefühl* [common senses]; see e.g. Heller-Roazen 2007; Paterson 2013).

A more sustained yet related objection was posed by fellow empiricist and near contemporary George Berkeley in 1709, recently echoed by J. L. Mackie (1976) and others, pointing out that Locke's answer contradicts his own renowned doctrine of so-called 'primary' and 'secondary' qualities of perception in the *Essay* (II.VIII). According to Cassirer, the entirety of Berkeley's *An Essay Towards a New Theory of Vision* (1709) was written as a response to Locke's treatment of the Molyneux problem. The rumination on the epistemological import of Locke's essay occupied Berkeley's mind, 'germinating cells from which his whole theory of perception developed', claims Cassirer, and Berkeley's essay 'is nothing but a complete systematic development and elucidation of Molyneux's problem' (1979: 109). Berkeley responds in part to the legacy of writers on optics, including Descartes' *Dioptrique* and Molyneux's *Dioptrica nova*, but offers a more empathetic and more philosophically cautious interrogation of hypothetical blind subjects:

> In order to disentangle our minds from whatever prejudices we may entertain with the relation to the subject in hand nothing is more apposite than the taking into our thoughts the case of one born blind, and afterwards, when grown up, made to see. And though perhaps it may not be an easy task to divest ourselves entirely of the experience received from sight so as to be able to put our thoughts exactly in the posture as such a one's: we must nevertheless, as far as possible, endeavour to frame true conceptions of what might reasonably be supposed to pass in his mind. (*Vision* §92)

Berkeley goes on to suggest that the subject would be uncertain whether anything was 'high or low, erect or inverted [...] for the objects to which he had hitherto used to apply the terms up and down, high and low, were such only as affected or were some way perceived by his touch; but the proper objects of vision make a new set of ideas, perfectly distinct and different from the former, and which can in no sort make themselves perceived by touch' (*Vision* §95). He therefore distinguishes carefully between sight and touch as ways of perceiving and knowing, and takes the position that it would take some time to learn to associate the two.

Prior to considering Berkeley's full response to the Molyneux question, we briefly summarise Locke's position on the perception of objects. Locke tells us that there is a crucial difference between two kinds of simple ideas we receive from sensation. Some resemble their causes out in the world, while others do not. The ideas that do resemble their causes, Locke argues, are ideas of 'primary qualities' such as texture, number, size, shape, motion. The ideas that do not resemble their causes are 'secondary qualities', the more subjectively sensed qualities of colour, sound, taste, and odour. Primary qualities exist in objects whether we perceive them or not, so Locke reasons that the ideas they cause in us resemble the bodies that cause them. The division between primary and secondary qualities leads to a strange amalgam of direct and indirect realism, whereby the primary qualities of objects exist independently of our perception of them. Conversely, the secondary qualities are dispositions or powers that objects have independently of experience, but they require perceivers for their sensory-based dispositions to be manifested, and do not resemble the actual qualities. As regards the Molyneux question, and following Martha Brandt Bolton's overview (1994: 79ff.) of Berkeley's objection to Locke, the difficulty is that 'shape-ideas' (primary qualities relating to the physical dimensions of an object perceivable to an observer) provide information about the features of their causes, the original object to be perceived. A cube causes both visual and tactile ideas of shape, for example, and if both visual and tactile ideas resemble the same cause (i.e. the cube), then Locke must allow some significant overlap between their contents. Since ideas of figure are directly perceived through both sight and touch, then, it is unclear what would stand in the way of the newly sighted man being able to recognise figures he sees for the first time as those previously felt. For Berkeley, Locke's doctrine of primary qualities is therefore inconsistent with his negative answer to the Molyneux question. Either Locke and Molyneux are incorrect, or else the sensations from sight are distinct from those of touch, and there is none of the overlap that Locke assumed. As Berkeley explains:

> Now, if a square surface perceived by touch be of the same sort with a square surface perceived by sight; it is certain the blind man here mentioned might know a square surface, as soon as he saw it. [...]

> We must therefore allow, either that visible extension and figures are specifically distinct from tangible extension and figures, or else, that the solution of this problem, given by those two thoughtful and ingenious men, is wrong. (*Vision* §133)

To retain consistency in developing his answer, Berkeley ends up rejecting Locke's system of primary and secondary qualities entirely, and argues for a negative answer to Molyneux's question for very different reasons to Locke and Molyneux, based on the radical incommensurability of sensations from sight and from touch, an explanation that eventually leads Berkeley to a metaphysical answer to Molyneux's problem based upon idealism. In the *Vision*, Berkeley's twist is that, in perceiving a cube, the specificity of tactile impressions is distinct from the specificity of visual sensations of that same cube, implying that there is no commensurability (cross-modal transfer) between vision and touch. Given that an object such as a cube or sphere has measurable dimensions, mass, and volume irrespective of their separate perceivable visible and tangible qualities, Berkeley poses the question 'whether the particular extensions, figures, and motions perceived by sight be of the same kind with the particular extensions, figures, and motions perceived by touch?' (*Vision* §127), then answers definitively: '*The extension, figures, and motions perceived by sight are specifically distinct from the ideas of touch called by the same names, nor is there any such thing as one idea or kind of idea common to both senses*' (*Vision* §127, original emphasis). Berkeley must be aware how counterintuitive this seems to the reader but, in a move familiar from Locke, he explains our multisensory experience of an object or an event as sheer coincidence, an habitual association of the data from one sense with that of another which fails to disprove his hypothesis of the ultimate incommensurability of the sensory modalities.

Furthermore, our judgement of the distance of such objects from the observer is not immediately derived from purely optical information but occurs in the mind (*Vision* §41–2), and is necessarily the result of previous separately channelled sensory experiences. In considering the measurement of distance and the way that objects have spatial extension, the question of the spatiality of perception and the perception of space becomes more prominent. Berkeley's refutation of Locke's answer to Molyneux rests not only upon his denial that cross-modal transfer between vision and touch is possible as a result of the divergence of the sensory modalities, but also crucially upon the rejection of any 'general' or abstract ideas whatsoever that might underlie such sensory input. Berkeley holds that there is no space common to all the senses, and no 'general' idea or innate concept of space (Morgan 1977: 179). The logical consequence is, rather bizarrely, that space is tactile rather than visual and hence there is no such thing as visual space. That spatial experience was predominantly a tactile phenomenon informs his approach to the original 1688 Molyneux question which, we remember, references the judgement of distance:

> From what hath been premised it is a manifest consequence that a man born blind, being made to see, would, at first, have no idea of distance by sight; the sun and stars, the remotest objects as well as the nearer, would all seem to be in his eye, or rather in his mind. The objects intromitted by sight would seem to him (as in truth they are) no other than a new set of thoughts or sensations, each whereof is as near to him as the perceptions of pain or pleasure, or the most inward passions of his soul. (*Vision* §41)

Berkeley's assumption about the complexities of spatial perception and the previously unconsidered issue of intercalating distance is prescient, since Cheselden's high-profile cataract operations remained decades away. Conventional wisdom would suggest, as does Locke, that each object we perceive, whether a cube or a sphere, would straightforwardly correlate one value for 'extension' (the three-dimensional volume of an object and its measurement in space) with one for 'figure' or shape. In Berkeley's words: 'But the extension and figure of a body, being let into the mind two ways, and that indifferently either by sight or touch, it seems to follow that we see the same extension and the same figure which we feel' (*Vision* §48). On further consideration this is not the case, and Berkeley talks us through his objection. For, despite conventional associations between sensations of touch and of vision in handling objects like cubes and spheres, say, still we must technically acknowledge that 'we never see and feel one and the same object' (*Vision* §49), because the visible values of extension and figures are perceived separately from tangible extension and figures (*Vision* §133). Here, the magnitude of the difference between Locke and Berkeley is revealed once again. Locke's 'ideas' are constituted as separate but related strands of sensory information, and given a shortfall in the data of one sense, blindness being an apt example here, there might still be in Locke's terminology the same 'general' (that is, abstract) idea of a cube or sphere that lies behind it. For Berkeley, since the data of sense are entirely separate and unrelated, this is categorically unthinkable.

Leibniz and Reid: blind man's geometry

Gottfried Wilhelm Leibniz also responded to Locke in his *Nouveaux essais*, written in 1704, and would have contributed more significantly to the debate had it not been for Locke's death that same year. Since the *Essais* involved an extended critical commentary on Locke and the Molyneux problem, Leibniz chose not to publish after Locke's death. They appeared in print posthumously in 1765, well after the initial wave of philosophical speculation on the matter, and without the benefit of post-operative evidence that later commentaries and contributions could offer. Nonetheless, Leibniz's positive answer to the Molyneux question is justified through rather unusual means. As an arch-rationalist, and having worked on logic and mathematics as well as philosophy, it is a little unexpected that he chooses not to invoke innate ideas in his justification that the Molyneux man would be able to identify the shapes of the cube and sphere immediately. As did Synge and Locke before him, Leibniz distinguished between 'images' that pertained to the senses and 'ideas' that consist of compounds of definitions. Likewise, images could be built up into more complex ideas, and while each image belonged to a particular sense, the more compounded idea that results belonged to 'the common sense, that is to say, the mind itself' (*Essais* II.IX.§8). Now, geometry relies on measures and proportions irrespective of how their depictions are manifested. An equilateral triangle is the same whether drawn on the sand, in a classroom, or modelled in clay, as geometry deals with compound ideas rather than images. Whether a person is blind, quadriplegic, illiterate, or mute, Leibniz would argue that each would arrive at the same geometry, with the same ideas irrespective of whether the images are tactile, visual, or auditory.

With such basic geometrical examples as a cube and a sphere, argues Leibniz, there are two notable implications. First, the Molyneux man is at an advantage in being told what objects they are beforehand, so merely chooses which is which. He need not identify the objects *ab initio*. Indeed, within Leibniz's rather idiosyncratic philosophy of mind it would be impossible to do so, as everyone is born with a complete set of ideas and the equipment for handling them. Our pre-given ideas are confused and must be ordered through empirical discovery, much as the patterns of veins in marble may be discerned only through working the material, thinks Leibniz (see Baxandall 1997: 20). According to Leibniz, then, the newly sighted Molyneux man would be able to distinguish the cube from the sphere but not instantaneously, as confusions would require resolution, and he would previously have needed tactile access to both objects. Secondly, whether a blind man uses tactile images or a quadriplegic only visual images, both would recognise that a sphere technically has no distinguishable points, whereas a cube has eight. Upon opening his eyes, the newly sighted man would count the distinguishable points via his visual image, rather than as previously through touch. As Leibniz explains in his chapter 'Of Perception':

> My view rests on the fact that in the case of the sphere there are no distinguished points on the surface of the sphere taken in itself, since everything there is uniform and without angles, whereas in the case of the cube there are eight points that are distinguished from all the others. If there weren't that way of recognising shapes, a blind man couldn't learn the rudiments of geometry by touch, nor could a sighted person learn them by sight without touch. However, we find that men born blind can learn geometry, and indeed always have some rudiments of a natural geometry; and we find that geometry is mostly learned by sight alone without employing touch, as must be done by a paralytic or by anyone else to whom touch is virtually denied. These two geometries, the blind man's and the paralytic's, must come together, and agree, and indeed basically rest on the same ideas, even though they have no images in common. (*Essais* II.IX.§8)

Leibniz's answer combines elements of Synge with more abstract reasoning based on geometry, something that would transpire in later answers to Molyneux by Hutcheson in his *An Essay on the Nature and Conduct of the Passions and Affections* (1728) and, for different reasons, by the Scottish philosopher Thomas Reid in *An Inquiry into the Human Mind on the Principles of Common Sense* (1764). Both rejected innate ideas and invoked ideas common to the senses, something supported by Locke through his concept of 'general' ideas. Leibniz's turn to geometry adds a fillip to the speculative reasoning around the Molyneux question by appealing to compound principles that are no longer limited to sensory presentation, to mathematical universals and geometrical abstraction rather than what our senses admit to perception. It is unclear from Leibniz's essays whether he knew of, or had met, Nicholas Saunderson, the blind Lucasian Professor of Mathematics at Cambridge. Saunderson invented a system of geometrical calculation using pegs on a wooden tabulated board that he could touch to determine answers. The blind mathematician was later celebrated by Reid and, notoriously, by Diderot in his *Lettre*. Such answers and contributions would extend the relevance of Locke's and Berkeley's responses since, as Riskin observes, 'both Locke and Molyneux shared with their opponents the assumption that the senses worked together to transmit whole impressions of a multifaceted external world' (2002: 25). Berkeley was excluded from this list due to the incommensurability of the sense modalities.

Later, Reid referred to post-operative vision in the *Inquiry* without directly alluding to Molyneux's question, but naming the Cheselden case. Space does not allow a detailed account of his views on the role of touch and vision in his larger epistemological project, but in a section of chapter six, entitled 'Of seeing', Reid suggests a useful separation between psychological and philosophical factors and holds a refreshingly sophisticated separation between visual phenomena, things as they appear to us and the newly sighted man, and more complex qualities that can be discerned only through experience and repeated exposure. Reid asserts:

> To a man newly made to see, the visible appearance of objects would be the same as to us; but he would see nothing at all of their real dimensions, as we do. He could form no conjecture, by means of his sight only, how many inches they were in length, breadth, or thickness. He could perceive little or nothing of their real figure; nor could he discern that this was a cube, that a sphere, that this was a cone, that a cylinder. (Reid 2000: 84–5)

Reid goes on to liken the visual experience of the newly sighted man to a person being exposed to an unknown language, who 'would attend to the signs, without knowing the signification of them' (2000: 85). Although this supplies a negative answer to Molyneux's question, throughout the book Reid consistently elides the difference between the blind and the sighted when it comes to matters of significance such as mathematics or astronomy, and recollections of ingenious demonstrations by Saunderson help him here. Indeed, section two of the chapter is entitled 'Sight discovers almost nothing which the blind may not comprehend', and he invokes the blind figure of Saunderson here and elsewhere to further solidify his argument in the *Inquiry* that concepts are independent of particular sensations (see e.g. Hopkins 2005). In that case, if knowledge can be acquired through non-visual means, why is Reid's answer to the Molyneux question negative? This is due to a distinction between what Reid later in the *Inquiry* terms 'original' and 'acquired' perception, which renders those immediate impressions on the eye less significant than other information such as depth, perspective, distance, and so on, qualities of extension discernible through touch:

> In all our senses, the acquired perceptions are many more than the original, especially in sight. By this sense we perceive originally the

visible figure and colour of bodies only, and their visible place: but we learn to perceive by the eye, almost every thing which we can perceive by touch. (2000: 171)

Notwithstanding Reid's negative answer to the Molyneux problem, his epistemological project is a development of Locke's. Corresponding to Locke's 'habitual custom', Reid suggests that through '[c]ustom, a sort of legerdemain' (2000: 167), the novelty and immediacy of visual sensations gradually recede in favour of those more dependable and informative physical qualities of objects that are anyway available to us through the means of touch. Thus, in Reid's terminology, we go from 'sensations' that directly correlate with objects in the world through the sense organs, to 'conceptions' where the mind is aware of the properties of those objects, and ultimately to 'perceptions' where we become aware of certain qualities of an object and a measure of certainty about this. While 'the excellence and dignity of this faculty' of sight (2000: 77) is noted, through its translation into 'conceptions' and then 'perceptions' we are ultimately left with the same kind of knowledge that a blind man like Saunderson has. Despite this more persistent knowledge having originally been generated through vision or touch, it becomes reducible to neither. For example, in holding a solid object like a ball, the tactile sensations are separable from the properties of the ball in terms of hardness, shape (figure), and size (extension): 'When I grasp a ball in my hand,' says Reid, 'I perceive it at once hard, figured and extended. The feeling is very simple, and hath not the least resemblance to any quality of body. Yet it suggests to us three primary qualities perfectly distinct from one another, as well as from the sensation which indicates them' (2000: 63).

This long and involved story in the wake of the Molyneux question has been more rigorously articulated in philosophical terms by Morgan in his *Molyneux's Question* (1977), and later Degenaar in her more historically oriented *Molyneux's Problem* (1996). In this chapter we have attempted something more modest, the introduction of a hypothetical epistemological problem for philosophy that implicates the particularity of perception through the modalities of touch and vision, and something of its historical context. But, in offering snapshots of responses in the wake of Molyneux by Berkeley, Synge, Leibniz, and Reid, we have been dancing around one of the core issues raised in the first place, one that underlies the potential translatability or otherwise between vision and touch for a blind subject: the types of knowledge available to us through touch and sight, and the possibility of more 'general' concepts that pertain to several senses at once.

We saw how Reid, for example, argued against the immediacy of visual sensation in favour of the more persistent abstract concepts dealing with extension, available to touch. A stated aim of Reid's *Inquiry* acknowledges this, involving extended discussions of the relationship between touch and sight, but also investigating whether there are what Hopkins in an essay on Reid terms 'common original perceptibles' (2005: 352), that is, things common to touch, vision, or indeed any sense modality. To inquire into the existence of such common perceptibles that underlie the sensations arising through particular modalities is to rejoin the stream of a philosophical discussion from Aristotle onwards, whether we term this common sensibles, common perceptibles, or a *sensus communis*.

Common sensibility and cross-modality: what Molyneux means for neonates

Unlike Berkeley, Descartes had never considered an abstract spatial framework through which we conduct geometrical and other calculations as tied to any sense modality. Even more unusually, touch was more originary than sight for Berkeley's concept of space. But if our concept of space were to subtract any sensory content, this entails an amodal spatial framework that diminishes the specific perceptual content of any of the different sense modalities. As a result, for both Descartes and Diderot, 'the senses are conceived more as adjuncts of a rational mind and less as physiological organs' (Crary 1990: 60). If the senses are merely rational adjuncts rather than distinct sensory modalities, what was at stake here in the possibility of cross-modal transfer, from touch to vision, hands to eyes? So far, we have argued through a series of nested philosophical debates. This concluding section briefly highlights the relevance of Molyneux's and Locke's legacy to some recent psychology literature, while remaining wary of imputing anachronistic views to historical figures. For example, for a modern instantiation of an amodal spatial framework, Lawrence Marks's fundamental 'unity of the senses' (1978) still references a unifying faculty at the cognitive level, much as Aristotle did through the *sensus communis* in *De anima* (424b–425a). This view still holds currency in some circles, for example Carreiras and Codina (1992). Yet, sagely enough, Diderot was actually arguing in the eighteenth century for something close to Graven's (2003) articulation of converging-diverging sensory subsystems and Gallagher's (2005) discussion of intermodal neonate vision.

According to the contemporary philosopher Naomi Eilan, answering 'yes' to Molyneux's question presumes 'that our perceptions are amodal in their spatial content' (1993: 237), a position for which she claims there is much empirical evidence, especially from child development studies. Piaget and Inhelder are well known for their empirical psychological approach to child development (e.g. 1956; 1969). Conversely, answering 'no' to Molyneux's question, as did Locke and Molyneux himself, is tantamount to arguing for the specificity of the senses, and what Eilan (1993: 240) describes as the 'radical incommensurability' of the different sensory systems. The Molyneux problem, translated into a more modern philosophical idiom, is therefore a true test of the limits and possibilities of cross-modal perception, but whether for a newly sighted man or in terms of neonatal development, this must be learned through forging and then repeating sensory associations, a systematic perceptual correlation that commences at birth for the sighted, or after the cataract operation for the congenitally blind. It relies on brain functions that are somewhat plastic and not yet narrowly specialised, even within the visual cortex. Renier et al., for example, in a study on cross-modal perception between audition and vision, show how 'some brain areas of the visual cortex are relatively multimodal and may be recruited for depth processing via a sense other than vision' (2005: 573). Accordingly, in chapter 7 we chart what happens to the visual cortex of a blind person learning Braille, considered as another form of sensory substitution, in this case of seeing with the fingers. In the wake of Molyneux, present to varying degrees in Locke through 'general' ideas, Reid, and others, perception across the modalities necessitates an abstracted, apprehending, unifying faculty or process that has the potential to transcend the immediacy of sensory experience, producing abstractions that may in some form be available subsequently to the other senses. Thus the sighted might perform the same mathematical calculations as the blind Nicholas Saunderson did through his wooden boards, pegs, and tables.

The role of the Molyneux question in the formation of a proto-psychology, or at least a psychologically complex philosophy that prepares the way for more sustained psychological inquiry, is threefold. First, being one of the persistent themes of this book, the assumption in folk psychology and also voiced by Descartes that the senses can be substituted, whether hands for eyes or touch for sight, fundamentally asks whether there is in some way an equivalence or, at least, translatability between the senses. If information is transferred from one sense modality to another, for example touch to vision, this is indeed a form of 'sensory substitution'. But we have considered whether the particularity of one modality (for example, the perception of texture in the fingers) equates in any straightforward way with another modality (for example, high-resolution images on the macula), and if so, whether this is not a *functional* equivalence between the senses, as opposed to an *absolute* equivalence. Moreover, what does this entail for brain functions if, as Descartes observed, we see with the mind rather than the eye, and the sense organs are mere adjuncts? Secondly, the Molyneux question remains unresolved to this day, despite the availability of post-operative evidence. Even recent philosophy and psychology literature (e.g. Evans 1985; Jacomuzzi et al. 2003; Gallagher 2005; Bruno and Mandelbaum 2010) addresses this problem, albeit with modified terms of reference. And thirdly, it directly questions the relevance of modern technologies of sensory substitution systems in positing the equivalence, or otherwise, of the senses, and in the case of vision and touch, of 'seeing with the hands' through electronic means.

Chapter 3

Objects that 'touch'd his eyes': Surgical Experiments in the Recovery of Vision

The man who learned how to see (but was disappointed with what he saw)

After fifty years of life as a blind person, at the age of fifty-two the Englishman Sidney Bradford attended a routine ophthalmic examination. These visits, which had been going on for several years, simply involved peering under the bandages he wore over his eyes. But this particular appointment turned out differently. Recent advances in surgical techniques meant that a graft could be performed to repair his corneal functioning. A corneal graft replaces the transparent surface of the eye with one from a donor. Such operations were becoming more readily available, and on 9 December 1958 Bradford underwent a corneal graft on his left eye; a month later his right eye was treated. After years of being classified as blind, being independent, and having set up home as a blind person, his sight was suddenly fully restored. The number of historical cases where ophthalmic surgery restores vision fully after complete blindness are exceptionally few and far between. A few weeks after the first graft, a report in the *Daily Express* about the successful surgery caught the eye of a laboratory assistant, Jean Wallace, and she informed her colleague Richard Gregory, then a lecturer in experimental psychology at Cambridge University. Dropping everything, and knowing Bradford's situation was time-sensitive, they drove to the hospital where he was being treated to begin a series of tests on him. The case study, known in the psychology literature through the anonymised moniker 'S.B.', became a *cause célèbre*. It launched Gregory's career, and boosted the study of the psychology of visual perception and the emerging interdisciplinary area known as 'vision science'. Descriptions of the surgery and its aftermath soon appeared in numerous psychology textbooks, which were routinely used by undergraduate students.

The resulting case study of S.B., written by Gregory and Wallace and published as a monograph in 1963, is salutary for a number of reasons. First, it is one of the most detailed psychological reports of sight restoration, a rare phenomenon that nonetheless had an illustrious history in medical reports and often engaged the public imagination. One of a series of intermittent reports spread throughout the centuries, there are clear commonalities with the celebrated first report to the Royal Society of a cataract operation on a teenage boy by the surgeon William Cheselden in 1728. Secondly, S.B. became a living incarnation of an empirical answer to the Molyneux problem, like Cheselden's patient, and raised the profile once again of this thorny epistemological issue within twentieth-century psychology literature. Thirdly, through close empirical observation of his interactions with objects and space, and through tests performed in the laboratory, the case of S.B. foregrounded the role of the brain and its adaptation within the visual system, as opposed to previous concentration on the functioning of the sense organs. S.B. became a living illustration of Descartes' prescient phrase from the sixth discourse of *Dioptrique* that 'it is the mind which sees, not the eye; and it can see immediately only through the intervention of the brain' (2001: 108). In fact, Gregory advanced his own succinct phrase as a result of S.B.'s case study that he later repeated elsewhere, including in *Eye and Brain* (1967). A blind man must 'learn how to see' all over again, thought Gregory, and 'the perceptual habits and strategies of touching and seeing' (Gregory and Wallace 1963: 37) over a lifetime must be changed, rethought, reconfigured. For an early-blinded adult, this means reversing the cortical plasticity and habits of perception that have resulted from a lifetime of adapting the visual cortex to non-optical tasks and specialisations, including heightened sensitivity to tactile and auditory perceptions. This cortical plasticity is more readily reversible at a young age, but having been operated on in later middle age, Bradford found it difficult to acclimatise fully to sight restoration. For a proportion of the miniscule number of subjects in history who have undergone ophthalmic surgery in order to see, the mismatch between the newly sighted world and the world previously familiar through touch is very great. Despite the best intentions of investigators like Gregory and his team, and Bradford's own wife and family, being one of the few people on the planet who, after complete blindness, had learned how to see, Bradford became 'The Man Who Was

Disappointed With What He Saw', in a memorable phrase from Claudia Hammond's BBC radio documentary about S.B. (2010). Flaky paint, dirty streets, and fast-moving cars all troubled him, he became clinically depressed, and he regressed into a world of darkness from which he never properly recovered. He died only two years after his restorative surgery. One of the foundational myths of the Enlightenment, the opening out on to a new visual order of truth and knowledge that Foucault had identified in *The Birth of the Clinic* (1963), was invested in the breathtaking promise of truly seeing the world for the first time, and an intensified dramatic anticipation of the removal of bandages before the light of truth. But this palled very quickly for Bradford. Just how did the 'truth' of seeing shift quite so markedly from the airy wondrousness of the Enlightenment ideal to the prosaic reality of streets and faces that disappointed in actuality? This chapter is the story of several case studies of sight restoration, although it distils common elements through the figure of S.B. in particular. Tellingly, there is a pattern in the case histories of learning to see, but being disappointed with what was seen.

If Cheselden's report is arguably the first genuine case study, other instances throughout history have occurred in written records. Marius von Senden's *Space and Sight* (1932, translated 1960) includes a historical review of cases of the recovery of vision, and mentions a few cases where depression or withdrawal ensued, and where previous tactile habits took over from acquired vision. Likewise, Alberto Valvo provided a historical survey in his *Sight Restoration after Long-Term Blindness* (1971). In the twentieth and twenty-first centuries, according to vision scientist Ione Fine (2009), other notable cases along with S.B. include T.G. and H.S. (Valvo 1971), H.B. (Ackroyd, Humphrey, and Warrington 1974), and more recently 'Virgil' (Sacks 1995), M.M. (Fine et al. 2003), and S.R.D. (Ostrovosky, Andalman, and Sinha 2006), the initials used in the scientific literature being standard practice to anonymise the research subject and protect privacy. All such cases, it turns out, confirm Gregory's observation that human subjects must 'learn' to see, and that without accumulating meaningful visual experience from which the brain can make sense of what the eyes see, merely having functioning eye organs is insufficient. Bradford's reaction differed greatly from that of Californian subject Michael May, who lost his sight aged three and recovered it forty years later. May was the subject of academic study (e.g. Fine et al. 2003) as well as an inspirational work of biography, *Crashing Through* (Kurson 2007).

However, von Senden's identification of a pattern of eventual withdrawal from the visual world by newly sighted subjects means that S.B.'s case is more typical. In historical accounts, the young musical prodigy Maria Theresia von Paradis coped with her blindness by testing various tactile writing technologies, which we will detail in chapter 6. Von Paradis reportedly had her blindness attended to, and possibly cured, by the influential and charismatic Franz Mesmer in 1777, after which she grew uneasy and reverted to her blind ways (Riskin 2002: 40). The recovery of vision after years of sight loss inevitably entails an emotional adjustment alongside any neurophysiological changes. The voluntary return to darkness, to the certainties and tactile truths of their pre-operative world, is telling, and clearly counters the Enlightenment narrative. The following section involves a case study from the psychology literature which examines post-operative vision and, since it includes several phenomena and features in common with other documented case studies, can be considered a distillation, exhibiting both Enlightenment narrative and counter-narrative, the freedom of vision followed by emotional withdrawal.

'Now that I've felt it, I can see': the case of S.B.

Born in Birmingham in 1906, the ten-month-old Sidney Bradford lost his sight in both eyes following an infection contracted after a smallpox vaccination. Thereafter he had weekly visits to an eye clinic to have his eyes examined and the bandages, which he had to wear routinely, replaced. As one of the psychology textbooks covering this case study reports, he was an independently minded man who had married and set up home (Rolls 2010). He would cross the road unaided, would usually not carry a white cane on his excursions, and was known to go on long bike rides, holding on to a friend's shoulder for guidance. His disposition was jovial, and he was competent with his tools as a cobbler. Gregory and Wallace arrived at the hospital some time after the corneal graft operation, but not long after Bradford's left eye had been first exposed to the light. In an article for *Nature* that summarised the impact of his original case study, Gregory judged him 'cheerful and confident' and, a useful trait for a research subject, 'truthful and honest' (Gregory 2004: 836). These brief biographical observations are noteworthy because of the dramatic change in Bradford's personality in the months following surgery, as he adjusted to a visual world and learned how to see. But what of the immediate aftermath of the unbandaging, that dramatic moment so fetishised by Cheselden and so resonant within the Enlightenment context, when he first opened his now-functioning eyes?

For any such case of a blind man being made to see, the first thing visually resolved is ordinarily the face of the surgeon, and Bradford was no different. According to the initial *Daily Express* article that prompted Gregory and Wallace's interest, Bradford said: 'I saw a dark shape with a bump sticking out and heard a voice, so I felt my nose and guessed the bump was a nose. Then I knew if this was a nose I was seeing a face' (Winn 1959: 7). Gregory twice in the monograph revisits the exact moment that Bradford had his bandages removed. First, paraphrasing Bradford's experience:

> He heard a voice coming from in front of him and to one side: he turned to the source of the sound, and saw a 'blur'. He realised that this must be a face. Upon careful questioning, he seemed to think that he would not have known that this was a face if he had not previously heard the voice and known that voices came from faces. (Gregory and Wallace 1963: 18)

Secondly, as part of a correspondence between Gregory, Marius von Senden, and the ophthalmic surgeon Hirtenstein that appears as an Appendix to Gregory and Wallace's monograph, Gregory clarifies this moment in a letter to von Senden: 'His account is that he heard Mr Hirtenstein's face and looking toward him (by Sound) "saw" a confusion of colours, and knew that this must be Mr. Hirtenstein's face' (Gregory and Wallace 1963: 42). However, certain observations about the first instances of vision after sight restoration proved to be provocative in the correspondence, prompting further letters for clarification from von Senden. These included, first: 'He was able, within hours, to name many objects correctly, and would get up early in the morning to watch cars passing on the street below' (1963: 42); and secondly, 'When the journalist of the *Daily Express* interviewed him Mr. B. told him with regard to his wife: "She was just as bonny as I thought she would be. My wife had given me a word picture of what the world was like and I found that the buses I travelled on and cars looked just as I imagined"' (1963: 39). This suggested a near instantaneous collocation between tactile, auditory, and visual sensations that was unlike anything von Senden had previously encountered in case studies of sight recovery, as he explained in his letter to Hirtenstein of 1959 (1963: 43). That initial *Daily Express* interview was followed by other stories on Bradford by the journalist but, naturally, none were scientifically rigorous. Bradford being reported as having instantaneous vision and declaring his wife to be 'bonny' was both diplomatic and sensationalised, for Gregory and Wallace reported that he had difficulty identifying faces for quite some time. This story of facial recognition after sight restoration echoes Michael May's first visual encounter with his wife, who he described as having 'bunched-up cheeks' (Kurson 2007: 130). Of course, from feeling his own face May understood that bunched-up cheeks indicated a smile, so from visual-tactile collocation knew that his wife was happy to see him: 'I can see you smiling' were among the first words May uttered after regaining his sight (Kurson 2007: 130). Apart from Bradford's more reserved disposition concerning his newly visual world, he exhibited unexpected behaviours in this post-operative state. Gregory and Wallace had travelled to Birmingham with a quantity of testing equipment and were keen to start collecting data, but upon arrival they were surprised to see Bradford already striding around the hospital corridors, opening doors without difficulty and passing through by correlating vision and touch.

At first it seemed that Bradford's sight was working normally, but it soon became clear that he retained the habits and behaviours of a blind man. He stared ahead in a fixed manner rather than shifting his gaze and scanning around the room, as sighted people do involuntarily. If his attention were brought to an object, he would fix upon and scrutinise it with heightened intensity, but he would fail to 'look' unless objects of interest were pointed out to him by others. In other words, he looked as he touched, with great focus and proximity, at objects such as lampposts, mirrors, and equipment. This is a common observation in such case studies. Valvo noted, for example, how T.G. attempted to learn the shapes of objects by searching for visual 'points of reference' that correlated with tactile memory: 'The real difficulty here is that simultaneous perception of objects is an unaccustomed way to those used to sequential perception through touch' (1971: 31). For the sighted, a visual scene seems instantaneous because of a series of oculomotor behaviours known as 'saccades' that are learned in early infancy (Burr and Morrone 2004). For those like Bradford with acquired vision in later life, there are patterns of 'looking' that include visual roaming, saccades, and selective focusing on objects as opposed to their backgrounds that never had the chance to develop fully.

A similar post-operative situation to Bradford's occurred in Oliver Sacks's case study 'Virgil', first published as the essay 'To see and not see' for *The New Yorker* magazine (1993), and then as a chapter with the same title in *An Anthropologist on Mars* (1995). Virgil is shown an apple but is unable to recognise it until he touches it. He is then shown a picture of an apple in a magazine, where he recognises the object but is unable to understand that he is seeing a picture rather than a real fruit. In a paper on Molyneux's problem that discusses Virgil's case, Jacomuzzi et al. question his confusion of two-dimensional pictorial surface and three-dimensional object: 'Is this happening because he has not yet learned appropriate associations between his haptic and visual experiences, or because the optics of his eyes and his oculomotor responses are still not fully functional?' (2003: 264–5). Such complex and acquired oculomotor behaviours are difficult to learn, yet they are crucial factors in any visual prosthesis, such as technologies of sensory substitution. This explains the lack of eye contact in one who now sees, which may have an uncanny effect on a sighted interlocutor.

It was an unassuming wall-mounted clock in Bradford's ward that provided the greatest shock for Gregory and Wallace. They realised that he could tell the time by simply looking at it. They tested out his abilities by setting the hands of a nurse's alarm clock at various positions, and Bradford was able to see the hands and tell the correct time. Being so recently and suddenly sighted, how had he achieved this? They assumed his prior expertise with touch was indispensable. As Gregory explains: 'Taking a large watch, which had no glass, from the top pocket of his jacket, he told its time by rapidly touching its hands, as he had done for many years. So he could see immediately, from earlier touch experience. At least for us, this was a turning point for understanding vision' (2004: 836). Needless to say, this was a perfect demonstration of cross-modal perception between touch and sight in a formerly blind subject. However, since the psychologists arrived in the wake of the operation and the unbandaging, and the journalist only made intermittent visits, they were unable to determine how long Bradford took to achieve this ability. The surprising observations about the watch were subsequently confirmed by Bradford's remarkable recognition of capital letters from a magazine that was lying nearby. At the blind school he had attended in Birmingham, it turned out, pupils were taught how to recognise upper-case letters through touch. Decades after the case study, Gregory wrote about its impact in psychology: 'Technically, Bradford showed cross-modal transfer from touch to vision, which no one knew about at that time, although it was soon discovered by other researchers studying primates' (2004: 836). Conversely, in other situations Bradford's newly acquired vision conflicted with his previously accrued tactile and auditory experiences. His situation therefore contrasted with the comparatively unformed youth of Cheselden's patient, who was a teenager of 13–14 years, which meant that when Gregory and Wallace conducted tests and exposed Bradford to optical illusions while he remained in hospital, the results were revealing.

Despite passing as sighted in his corridor-wandering and day-to-day activities, Bradford's test results were far from normal. The well-known Necker cube is comprised of the outlines of two connected squares on paper. For sighted subjects the illusion is of a three-dimensional square whose surfaces can flip in orientation back and forth, so that the 'nearest' square surface can become the 'furthest' surface and *vice versa*. Cheselden's patient had initially had difficulty resolving patches of colour into representations of objects, and consequently with the conversion of two-dimensional representations into three-dimensional perspective. Bradford had real difficulty with the Necker cube's ambiguity and similar illusions involving dynamic changes in appearance, as 'pictures looked flat and meaningless' to him (Gregory 2004: 836). Titchener circles are visual illusions that check for the perception of size constancy, with two same-sized circles surrounded by other circles. The circle appears smaller when surrounded by larger circles, and larger when surrounded by smaller ones. These illusions work by drawing in contextual information from previous sighted experience, so small children have a different response to that of adults. Since Bradford was unable to reference previous sighted experience, not only did he fail to see the Necker cube as three-dimensional, he also failed to see the Titchener circles as different sizes. In the Zollner illusion he failed to see the vertical lines as slanted, as normal adult vision would. One might say this was literally 'unadulterated' vision, uninformed as it was by the rules and conventions that accrue from prior visual experience, including perspective. Since pictures looked flat to Bradford, perspective was not processed in his visual system, and since he could not detect interposition, he was not able to judge that one object was nearer than another because it overlaid or blocked the view of another.

However, it would be a mistake to straightforwardly equate Bradford's visual development with that of infants. Hitherto, the assumption in psychology was that there would be such parallels between the newly sighted and neonates; such, for example, was the view of T. K. Abbott in 1864 and William James in 1890. Likewise, the redoubtable twentieth-century Canadian psychologist Donald Hebb considered sight to be acquired only slowly and gradually in his hugely influential *The Organization of Behavior* (1949). In a section of the book that appraises historical cases of recovery after blindness, Hebb claimed: 'We are not used to thinking of a single perception as slowly and painfully learned, [...] but it has already been seen, in the discussion of the congenitally blind after operation, that it actually is' (1949: 77–8). This is not quite true, Gregory argues (2004), since evidence that face detection occurs merely hours after birth in humans reveals that the visual system is functional and responds to visual stimuli at a very early stage. Of course, it is not the fully developed visual system that recognises whole scenes or illusions, so it could still be claimed after Hebb, and is confirmed in Bradford's case, that sight is almost instantaneous but that visual learning, the process of learning to see that includes perspective and the ability to recognise illusions, is indeed more gradual. Bradford's situation was not that he was learning slowly from scratch, as would a neonate. Instead, his prior exposure to richly tactile experiences was informing his perceptions and, in some cases, had to be unlearned. Two brief examples demonstrate this.

First, perspective. While two-dimensional pictures ordinarily looked flat to him, for those objects that were already familiar from touch, such as chairs and tables scattered around his hospital ward, Bradford could judge distances and sizes. Earlier haptic explorations and walking experiences somehow calibrated his newly visual sense. But for pictures or untouchable objects his vision proved useless and, in some cases, positively dangerous. Bradford's judgement of scale, distance, and perspective was remarkably inaccurate, and this falls into line with other newly sighted subjects, including Cheselden's patient. Looking down from a high window on to the street, Bradford experienced a 'marked scale distortion' whereby he misjudged the distance and thought he could climb down 30–40 feet with his hands (Gregory and Wallace 1963: 18). When he later saw the position of the window from the street below, he realised his error of judgement.

Secondly, mirrors. Gregory and Wallace reported Bradford being fascinated with the optical effect of mirrors, and at first he found it difficult to believe that he could not reach out and touch a person reflected in one. This phenomenon is presumably aligned with the perception of the two-dimensional pictorial surface. Mirrors continued to exert a pull on Bradford's consciousness for quite some time. Soon after being discharged from hospital he stayed in a London hotel to meet Gregory for follow-up interviews and tests, and chose to sit facing a large wall mirror so he could see the entire room. Likewise, a year later, his favourite place to sit was near a mirror which afforded a view of the street outside (Gregory and Wallace 1963: 30). The nature of this fascination with mirrors is different from Cheselden's patient proclaiming that it seemed that objects 'touch'd his eyes', but Diderot reported from his interviews that a blind man in Puiseaux had 'often spoken of mirrors' (Diderot 1916a: 71). It is possible to infer from this that the fascination exerted on Bradford by mirrors was produced, at least in part, by the distinctly visual properties of an object that benefited little from his prior tactile experience, that extended his visual abilities purely through optical means, and which presented distinguishable objects to him that were nonetheless resolvable and recognisable. This fascination with mirrors continued for six months after the operation, Gregory and Wallace noted, and quite possibly thereafter.

Some weeks after the operation, Gregory took Bradford around some tourist sites in London. Strangely, he showed little interest in the scenery as they travelled, and there were signs that he had become jaded by novel visual encounters, and he complained to Gregory that the world seemed like a 'drab place' (Gregory and Wallace 1963: 30). This was the beginning of a long, slow descent. After much effort to acclimatise to his newly visual world, Bradford started to become disappointed with what he saw; the flaky paint and dirty streets did not correlate with his prior visual imagination, and he became clinically depressed. Cars terrified him. In contrast to Michael May, the Californian recipient of stem cell treatment which recovered his vision, Bradford's suffering may have derived from a misplaced optimism about what the sighted world was actually like, an optimism that was peeled away layer by layer after every successive day as a sighted man:

> Bradford said that he had expected to see a more perfect place when his bandages came off, that he had always imagined the sighted world as a kind of heaven. Now he knew it was less than that. He could see it in the frayed wood and stained fabrics and smudged windows he encountered daily, that no matter which way he turned things fell short of what he'd hoped they would be. He could see the truth in chipped paint and it disappointed him. (Kurson 2007: 87)

As a fully blind man, if Bradford wanted to cross the road he would simply stick out his white cane, march across the street, and cars would slow down for him. As a newly sighted man, however, he became terrified at the sight of cars speeding around, and was incapable of crossing the road unless dragged across by helpers. Gregory described the heart-breaking change from a fully functioning blind man to a half-disabled sighted man in Hammond's radio documentary (2010). Although the London visit revealed disappointments, nevertheless certain moments captivated Bradford's attention. Most telling was his reaction to a Maudesley screw-cutting lathe from around 1800 in the Science Museum, an object he could comprehend through his previous tactile interactions with tools and equipment in his shed, and his job mending shoes. Like most museum objects it was kept out of reach, in a glass case, but Bradford asked an attendant to open the case and was granted direct access. Bradford became much more involved with the object, manually exploring the machine to determine the individual parts. As Gregory and Wallace describe, the effect was startling: 'He ran his hands eagerly over the lathe, with his eyes tight shut. Then he stood back a little and opened his eyes and said: "Now that I've felt it I can see"' (1963: 31). Despite the rich visual nature of his visit to the tourist sites after his lifetime of blindness, it was the promise of correlating his tactile experience with his new visual abilities that most impressed him.

With regard to the visual illusions, the erroneous judgements about scale and perspective, and possibly his fascination with mirrors, the evidence suggests that his spatial reference frame was affected by his newly functioning 'unadulterated' visual abilities, and that when prior tactile experience could not be invoked errors of judgement were rife. Or, in Gregory's words: 'His unusual responses to the figures suggested that many illusions result from cognitive processing, rather than physiological signal processing occurring early in the visual system; this led to experiments and interesting controversies that persist today' (2004: 836). These words might remind us of Descartes' refrain from a less scientifically sophisticated but equally inquisitive age, 'it is the mind which sees, not the eye'. In S.B., the reverberations of this refrain were felt in the psychology of vision, and the import of cross-modal perception was truly established. Now we return to a time just after Molyneux's question, and the first documented case study of the restoration of vision.

Cheselden's patient

At the time Molyneux's question was initially posed to Locke in 1688, very little empirical evidence existed, mainly due to the fact that cataract operations were not routine, not always successful, not always reported, and sometimes faked. It would be almost forty years before the surgeon William Cheselden reported the case of an unnamed boy of around thirteen who gained his sight after the removal of lenses rendered opaque by cataract. His report to the Royal Society, published in the *Philosophical Transactions of the Royal Society* in 1728, was rather breathlessly entitled in full 'An account of some observations made by a young gentleman, who was born blind, or who lost his sight so early, that he had no remembrance of ever having seen, and was couch'd between 13 and 14 years of age'. His boy patient, with undetermined levels of pre-operative vision, had great difficulty interpreting aspects of the visual world, especially scale and perspective. In the report Cheselden noted: 'When he first saw, he was so far from making any Judgment about Distances, that he thought all Objects whatever touch'd his Eyes (as he express'd it)' (1728: 448).

Cheselden's surgery was by no means the first successful case, as there was a long tradition of the 'couching' of cataracts. The historical record is sporadic and difficult to verify, but points to precedents for these ophthalmic interventions centuries earlier. The psychologist Marius von Senden charts the history of successful 'couching' of cataracts in the Middle East in 1020, an operation on a man of thirty, although the details are vague and the source unverified (von Senden 1960; also Gregory and Wallace 1963). Other records go further back to India, where the physician Sushruta described the operation in the sixth century. Couching was a primitive but often effective technique in which thin needles were inserted into the eye to detach the clouded lens from the pupil, thereby readmitting light, a technique that was subsequently introduced from India into China and the Middle East (Finger 1994: 70). More recently, archaeological finds from Roman Britain of specialised couching needles known as *specilla*, along with a written account by the Roman author Celsus of the Alexandrian school who described the process of couching in AD 29, support the view that a range of eye conditions and diseases were treated as part of a long-running healthcare practice that addressed spiritual as well as physical aspects through a mixture of medicines, surgery, and votive offerings to the gods (Summerton 2008: 40).

Closer to the period of the Molyneux question, the reports become less sporadic and more frequent. Other cases of sight restoration were reported in 1668, 1695, 1704, and 1709, and since the Cheselden case of 1728 there have apparently been upwards of fifty reported cases (Gregory and Wallace 1963: 5), although Alberto Valvo (1971) offers the more conservative estimate that less than twenty cases have been known in the last 1,000 years. Cheselden's report to the Royal Society in London of 1728 was the most celebrated and became a sensation both in Britain and abroad, attracting widespread interest and credibility. It was subsequently discussed in France by Diderot, Buffon, Condillac, and Voltaire. Voltaire introduced a French readership to Cheselden's case study in his work of popular science *Elements of Newton's Philosophy*, published in 1738, and the sudden French interest in Cheselden's surgical experiments is the principal subject of the next chapter. Here, in evaluating the legacy of Cheselden's surgery, we consider how the newly available surgical evidence prompts questions about blindness and 'learning to see' that astonishingly continue to be asked through case studies into the twentieth and twenty-first centuries. These questions include the role of the senses in spatial perception by the blind, the experimental observations of cross-modal transfer, and parallels between infant development and the process of 'learning to see' in newly sighted adults. During this journey through experiments in ophthalmic medicine, early psychology, and philosophical speculation, however, new ways of conceptualising experiences of blindness are thrown up, and more sophisticated questions concerning the mechanisms of vision and of 'learning to see' are asked.

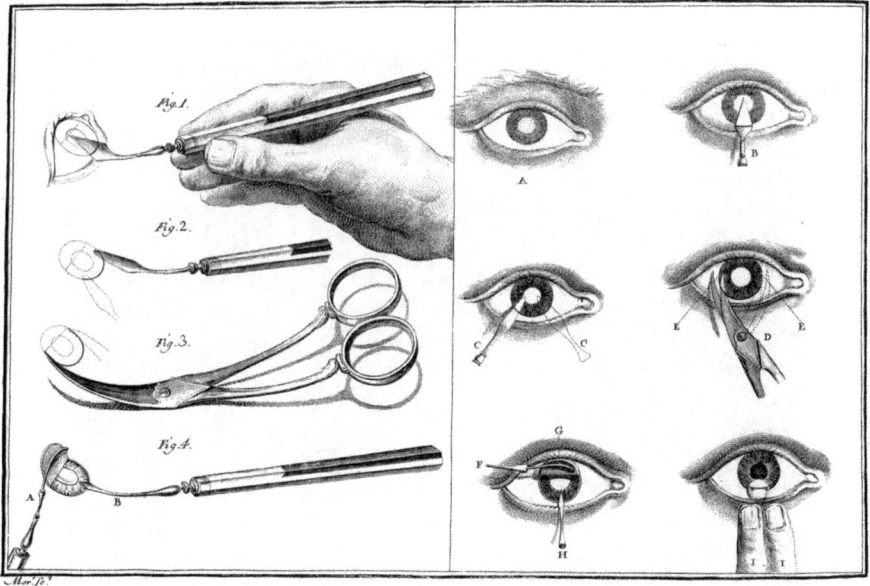

Figure 3.1 Instruments used in cataract operations. From a 1780 edition of Johannes de Gorter's *Cirugia Expurgada*.

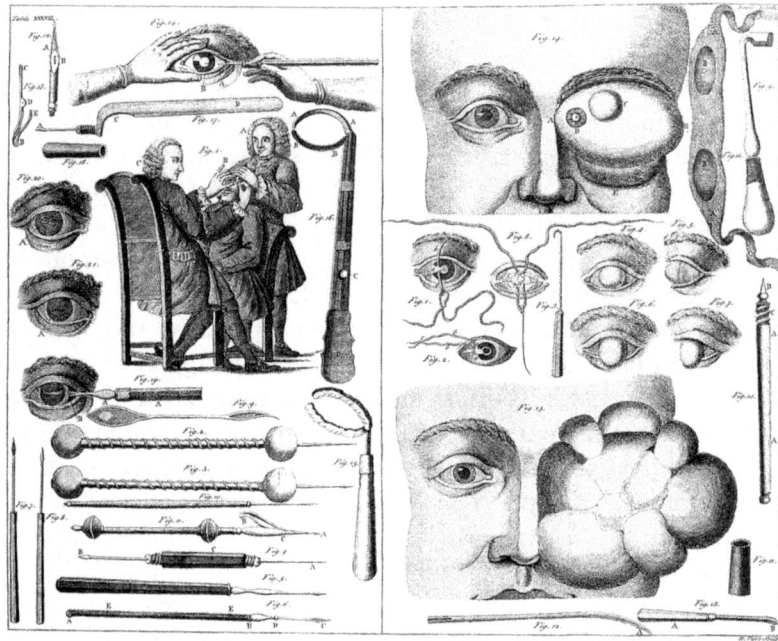

Figure 3.2 A double sheet showing various ophthalmology instruments, eye growths, a cataract operation, and other eye defects. Line engraving by R. Parr, 1743–45.

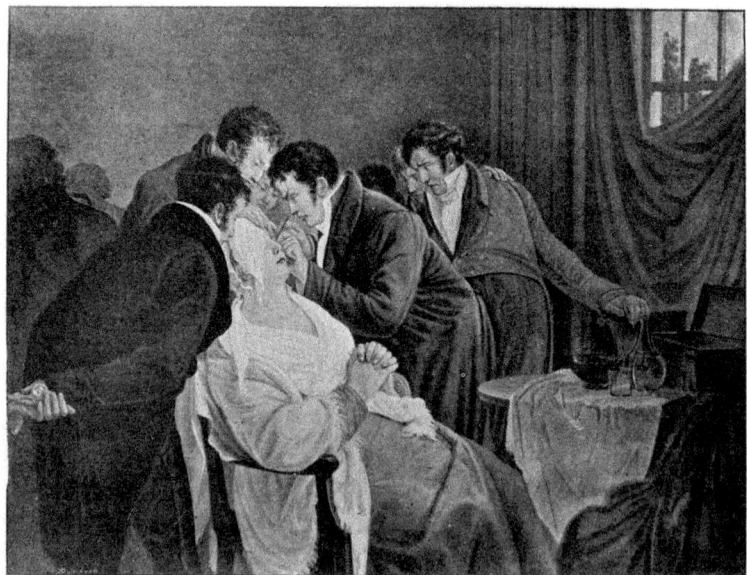

Figure 3.3 Guillaume Dupuytren operating on a cataract, source unknown.

Berkeley was the first to grasp the potential of experiences of the recovery of vision after blindness as a solution to Molyneux's problem. In the Appendix to the second edition of his *Essay Towards a New Theory of Vision* of 1710 he wrote that, shortly after the publication of the first edition in 1709, a case of a twenty-year-old man born blind who had undergone surgery to recover his sight had become known to him. His *Essay*, as we saw, was written partly in answer to Locke's treatment of Molyneux's problem and advanced the cause of empiricism, essentially claiming that there is no necessary connection between the visual field and the sensations of touch, and that any connection between those modalities could be established only through experience. In the Appendix to the second edition, having acknowledged that this recent example of the recovery of vision might contribute to the debate, Berkeley thus set a challenge to his reader:

> Such a one may be supposed a proper judge to decide how far some tenets laid down in several places of the foregoing essay are agreeable to truth, and if any curious person hath the opportunity of making proper interrogatories to him thereon, I should gladly see my notions either amended or confirmed by experience. (Berkeley 1975: 59)

In fact this was a celebrated case, reported by Robert Steele in his respectable London periodical of ideas and letters, *The Tatler*, in 1709. The operation in question had been performed by Roger Grant, a self-styled 'oculist' with no formal training who was soon regarded as a fraud, and the story discredited. Steele's report in *The Tatler* is rather melodramatic and overblown, and the standard components of these accounts, including the tense and emotionally heightened moments after the operation of recognising his mother and then his lover through their voices, are conveyed in overly sentimental language. At times the account has some semblance of truth: 'When the patient first received the dawn of light, there appeared such an ecstasy in his action, that he seemed ready to swoon away in the surprise of joy and wonder. The surgeon stood before him with his instruments in his hand. The young man observed him from head to foot…', at which point the patient considers the surgical instruments as extensions of the surgeon's hands (Steele 1898: 45). After emotional exchanges with his loved ones he is then urged to put bandages on to recover further, at which point the reader is left in little doubt that this was far from responsible ophthalmic practice. Steele's report then descends into saccharine exchanges between the lovers about visual beauty and the nature of love before the bandages are removed once and for all, in a final melodramatic flourish. Both Berkeley and London society were temporarily hoodwinked by a showman, it turned out, who was a part-time Baptist preacher and former cobbler, and who most probably made poor vision even worse on an untold number of patients through unskilled ocular surgery (see Steele 1898: n. 1; Degenaar 1996). Understandably, Berkeley never referred to Grant's operation again, but he did take notice of Cheselden's later published report in 1728, summarising its most significant points in *The Theory of Vision Vindicated and Explained* (1733).

While technically not the first cataract operation, as we saw, Cheselden's remained the most celebrated and widely reported example of a procedure that Berkeley and others recognised as having the potential to resolve the Molyneux question. Cheselden's detailed description had a greater impact than Grant's, as his reputation as a surgeon was by then established both in England and abroad. In fact Cheselden's reputation spread so far and wide that Condillac specifically mentioned the report as evidence for a coordinating function between the senses (Jütte 2005: 133), and Voltaire, who never met Cheselden, noted that he was 'one of those famous Surgeons, who unite a great Extent of Knowledge with Dexterity in Operations' (1991: 63–4). Unlike Grant, Cheselden was no charlatan or opportunist, being the author of the first English textbook on anatomy, and as an assistant surgeon in a series of London hospitals, he was influential in establishing surgery as a properly scientific medical profession. Hitherto, surgeons had been treated as glorified butchers, even using the same tools as barbers, so Cheselden's membership of the London Company of Barber-Surgeons in 1710 was testament to this new-found respectability. He had a role in the subsequent separation of surgeons from barbers, and the creation of the independent Company of Surgeons in 1745, which later became the Royal College of Surgeons. Surgery was snobbishly seen as a manual skill, or as Roy Porter puts it, a 'cutter's art' (2003: 115), compared to the professional competence of the physician, but the rise of more efficient techniques such as Cheselden's excision of bladder stones in minutes rather than hours, and the necessity for military surgeons to treat gunshot wounds, accelerated the acceptability of surgery, as Porter describes in his history of medicine (2003: 115–17).

Opthalmic surgery was another of Cheselden's strengths, of course. Prior to the famous cataract surgery, Cheselden knew little of his unnamed patient apart from the fact that the boy was between thirteen and fourteen years of age, and that the blindness was not total, meaning the boy had sensitivity to light and perhaps to colour, but certainly no ability to discern the shape of an object. In this way, says Cheselden with an arresting turn of phrase in his report to the Royal Society, 'they can discern in no other Manner, than a found Eye can through a Glass of broken Jelly' (1728: 447), implying that light rays could not be focused in order to resolve into their specific shapes within the eye. This type of blindness was common in cataracts, where light perception exists but no images can be resolved. The report continues:

> Tho' we say of the Gentleman that he was blind, as we do of all People who have Ripe Cataracts, yet they are never so blind from that Cause, but that they can discern Day from Night; and for the most Part in a strong Light, distinguish Black, White, and Scarlet; but they cannot perceive the Shape of any thing [...] wherefore the Shape of an Object in such a Case, cannot be at all discern'd, tho' the Colour may. (1728: 447)

Naturally, shortly after surgery Cheselden performed tests to determine the level of vision his patient now experienced, and what could be discriminated in terms of shapes and colours. Initially the distances, sizes, and shapes of objects could not be differentiated and, in line with Locke's argument concerning two-dimensional paintings and the necessity of learning how to see them as three-dimensional shaded objects, it was months before pictures of objects were understood not as the objects themselves but as representations. Cheselden's record of the aftermath of the operation is neither as systematic nor as consistent in detail as would be expected today, but some of his observations remain insightful, and not just for medical scholars. In that critical moment of unbandaging after the cataracts were removed, despite his youth and purported intelligence, Cheselden's patient found the simplest visual perceptions difficult and demonstrated no awareness of distance, size, or space. Cheselden reports:

> When he first saw, he was so far from making any Judgment about Distances, that he thought all Objects whatever touch'd his Eyes (as he express'd it) [...] He knew not the Shape of any thing, nor any one thing from another, however different in shape, or Magnitude; but upon being told what Things were, whose Form he before knew from feeling, he would carefully observe, that he might know them again. (1728: 448)

What Cheselden describes here is an interactive version of the Molyneux problem that he conducted with the patient shortly after the operation. Instead of recognising the differentiation only of a cube and a sphere, Cheselden's patient was given the task of perceiving and identifying a range of objects, including most notably a dog and a cat. Given the blurry nature of the presumably similarly sized furry exemplars that stood before him, the patient could be forgiven for being confused as to which was which. 'Having often forgot which was the Cat, and which the Dog, he was asham'd to ask; but catching the Cat (which he knew by feeling) he was observed to look at her steadfastly, and then setting her down, said, So Puss! I shall know you another time', reported Cheselden (1728: 448). The full title of the report unequivocally refers to the boy as having been 'born blind', and having 'no remembrance of ever having seen', yet by acknowledging sensitivity to light level and perhaps to colour earlier within his text, Chiselden questions the nature and extent of the subject's previous visual experience. Consequently, it is difficult to gauge the level of shape recognition the patient enjoyed before and indeed after the operation, and in addition the overall level of visual acuity before and after the operation remains imprecise and largely unquestioned. Consequently, Cheselden's account is rather limited in utility, being brief, unscientific, unstructured, and primarily anecdotal. By not including a sustained comparison between the patient's perceptual abilities before and after the operation, it further mystifies the degree and nature of the patient's experience and level of blindness and therefore limits any rounded assessment of the operation's effectiveness. In describing the task of differentiating the cat from the dog, for example, the wording provides only a rudimentary sense of the progressive capacities of the patient's visual perception after the operation. More pertinently here, neither does it definitively answer the Molyneux problem, since it perpetuates uncertainties concerning the patient's perception of objects before and after the cataract operation. And yet there are brief but intriguing echoes of more complex emotional issues that would become recognised in psychological and autobiographical accounts of blindness much later in the twentieth century, including that of Sidney Bradford. Furthermore, one passage directly addresses the issue found in Locke's *Essay Concerning Human Understanding* about paintings and two-dimensional representations of solid objects.

Showing pictorial representations of objects to the newly sighted patient, Cheselden at first assumed he could see the objects depicted. Instead, the patient initially saw them as coloured surfaces and nothing more. In Cheselden's words, the patient 'consider'd them only as Party-coloured Planes, or Surfaces diversified with Variety of Paint' (1728: 449), that is, as variously coloured surfaces. Initially at least, he effectively demonstrated what Berkeley, not Locke, considered the

Molyneux man might do after regaining sight. If Berkeley was correct, the separate data from touch and sight were incommensurable, and there would be no way of determining that a pictorial representation of an object 'looked' suitably solid and three-dimensional unless there was active correlation between those senses. Through touch alone, a sightless person would perceive the picture as a flattish surface with minimal marks or indentations, and through sight alone merely as an indeterminable pattern of shades, patterns, and colours. If Berkeley were correct then only through prolonged tactile and visual activity would the subject start to correlate information from these incommensurable modalities to produce a suitably tactile-visual object occupying three-dimensional space. But most likely the collective perception of the object would remain as a minimally three-dimensional object (the picture and frame), as opposed to further perceiving the patterns on its surface as representations of fully realised multi-dimensional objects. Conversely, Locke had not only argued for the habitual association of the senses as we have seen through his 'ideas', but in arguing for the possibility of 'abstract ideas' he allowed ideas that are non-specific to any particular sense modality within the cognitive faculty of the understanding, entailing the possibility of cross-modal transfer. The sighted subject would almost immediately, in effect, be able to intuit from past visual-tactile experience that the marks, shades, and patterns of pictorial representations were indexical, referring to the qualities of three-dimensional objects despite their being two-dimensional in composition.

Two months later, something unexpected and intriguing happened. Cheselden's patient had suddenly learned to see tactile properties within pictorial representations, implying that cross-modal perception was taking place. If this were the result of a Lockean abstract idea it would most probably have happened immediately, or at least sooner. In discovering that the 'Party-coloured Planes' were not just surfaces but 'represented solid Bodies' (1728: 449), had Cheselden's patient, in effect, confirmed Berkeley's hypothetical position? Having undergone this perceptual transformation, akin to resolving figure from ground for the Gestaltists, it might therefore seem counterintuitive that, on reaching out to touch the pictorial surface, the surface remained a flat plane rather than having the three-dimensional quality that his eyes had learned to see. As Cheselden put it, 'even then, he was no less surpriz'd, expecting the Pictures would feel like the Things they represented, and was amaz'd when he found those Parts, which by their Light and Shadow appear'd now round and uneven, felt only flat like the rest' (1728: 449). The visual system, having only recently acquired rules of perspective and the conventions of shade and colour gradation in the perception of material objects, is nonetheless fooled by how this can be achieved on a two-dimensional surface. In his somewhat confused and befuddled state, Cheselden's patient reportedly then asked the surgeon 'which was the lying Sense, Feeling, or Seeing?' (1728: 449). In other words, soon after cataract surgery the patient demonstrates cross-modal transfer in his recognition of forms and shapes, although not in the case of the dog and cat. But in the perception of pictorial representation his cross-modal transfers falter. As time progresses, ever more diverse sets of visual properties become perceptible, including the qualities of size and shape of previously untouched objects, and so the business of correlating newly acquired visual information with previous tactile information continues apace. But in this post-operative sensory flux, Cheselden's patient asks his question about the lying senses in earnest, as the need for verification requires that one sensory modality be the reference point for other sensory information. This might imply, even if temporarily, an implicit hierarchy of the senses in order to resolve visual figure from tactile ground in cases of indeterminacy or doubt. Further surgical experiments and epistemological speculations would continue to explore the unfolding of the post-operative relationship between touch and vision right through to the twentieth and twenty-first centuries, as we shall see, but along the way the accounts become more systematic, and some focus on the role of the senses in the psychology of spatial perception by the blind. The next section offers some highlights in the psychology and philosophy literature in the wake of Cheselden.

After Cheselden: psychological inquiry into spatial perception after the recovery of sight

In 1864 an Irish philosopher called Thomas Abbott published a book whose purpose was to challenge fellow Irishman Berkeley's ideas of touch and vision. Its title was certainly honest in intent, being *Sight and Touch: An Attempt to Disprove the Received (or Berkleian) Theory of Vision*. Early in the twentieth century, Abbott published an essay in the hugely respected journal *Mind* which reflected once again upon the significance of Cheselden's operation for the Molyneux problem, especially in light of other operations that had followed in the nineteenth century. Considering Molyneux's thought experiment within the context of developments in medicine and a more rigorous empirical psychology, towards the beginning Abbott attempts to place us almost empathetically within the mind of the Molyneux man. 'It is no doubt very difficult, perhaps impossible, for us with our life-long habit of visualising absent objects, or those which we handle in the dark, or with shut eyes, to put ourselves in the position of one who on first acquiring sight has to reproduce in imagination a tactual perception,' writes Abbott. He continues: 'Nevertheless it is not unreasonable to expect that in the case supposed the subject of the experiment would be able to discriminate correctly between the two figures' (1904: 544).

Answering the Molyneux question in the affirmative was nothing new in itself, but Abbott's contribution to the scholarship lies in his advancing Leibniz's answer, which concerned the perception of geometrical shape underlying the sensory modalities, in the light of more contemporary findings in vision science and physiology. To recap, Leibniz's answer was written in 1704 but published posthumously in 1765, and suggested that the smooth surface of the sphere would be visibly uniform from a number of different angles, whereas the cube's corners would be visible and in fact multiply when the head moves around the object. Abbott constructed an original and plausible rationale for his affirmative answer based on the visual perception of geometric shape alongside the muscle movement of the eye. In other words, the answer now involves a wider notion of visual perception that includes movement of the muscles surrounding the eye in order to direct the eye's orientation, a process known as oculomotor (or sometimes ocular-motor) perception. Eye movement is continual and forms a large part of visuo-spatial perception, so that instead of moving our entire heads around to apprehend a room and the objects within it, eye movements known as saccades help to continually fill in visual information to gauge depth, dimensions, and aid interaction with objects and the performance of tasks. Whereas this psychophysiological explanation for everyday perception was not part of the philosophical vocabulary of Molyneux or Leibniz, the famous Victorian philosopher J. S. Mill had argued that the perception of an object's spatial extension involved movements of the eye and therefore, in Abbott's words, 'a succession of muscular sensations', where the eye tracks or follows the shape of an object when apprehending it; the visual perception of a circle, for example, would consist of 'the consciousness of a series of eye movements' (Abbott 1904: 545 n. 1). For the eye to perceive a circle it would travel around the outline or figure of the circle, and 'it does so in a uniform manner and without check or interruption whereas in the case of the square there is an abrupt change of direction, and this might be expected to recall the change experienced by touch' (Abbott 1904: 545). This is an intriguing development. In the Molyneux situation the figures of sphere and cube apprehended in this way should be markedly different enough to at least determine which of the two is the sphere, especially if some movement of the head or eyes is permitted after the operation. In this Abbott also partly follows a Dr Jurin, quoted in Smith's *A Compleat System of Optics* of 1738, who assumes that any newly sighted Molyneux man must be at liberty to view figures and shapes from all sides and perspectives. In so doing they would find that the sphere always presents the same aspect, whereas the cube is more various.

In 1839 the doctor J. C. A. Franz's treatise on *The Eye* had also suggested an affirmative answer to Molyneux's question in a way that is consistent with both Leibniz and Jurin. Writing about the Molyneux man, Franz reasons: 'The supposed person will certainly be able to distinguish by his sight the cube from the sphere, though he will not, it is true, recognise the two figures as a *cube* and a *sphere*, but will pronounce the one to be a disc and the other a square.' He qualifies his answer, however, with the crucial consideration of the post-operative process, one that factors in the difficult adjustment to vision: 'it must be premised, however, that some little time must be allowed for the mind to recover from the confused sensation produced by the novelty and multitude of objects suddenly presented to the newly acquired faculty' (1839: 32).

Later, William James's *The Principles of Psychology* of 1890 considered Cheselden's post-operative text in order to ruminate on illusions of distance perception in children and adults, the most outstanding feature for him being the tactile illusion that distant objects form proximal impressions, have actual contact, and therefore seem to touch the eyes. James uses the striking simplicity of this fundamental perceptual error to further analogise between the experiences of the newly sighted subject and the development of perceptual laws and correlations that occur in child development. Whether or not James was the first to explicitly tie these observations about post-operative vision to the development of the visual system in infants, later experimental psychologists such as Gregory (1967) and Jacomuzzi et al. (2003), and philosophers of perception including Eilan (1993), have assumed this association to be commonplace. Echoing almost exactly the expression of Cheselden's patient that objects 'touch'd the eyes', James makes the connection here with the development of perception in infants:

> And other patients born blind, but relieved by surgical operation, have been described as bringing their hand close to their eyes to feel for the objects which they at first saw, and only gradually stretching

out their hand when they found that no contact occurred. Many have concluded from these facts that our earliest visual objects must seem in immediate contact with our eyes. (1927: 36–7)

Distance perception in small children, James reasons, must occur through the trial and error process of realising that objects do not, as Cheselden's patient described, in fact touch the eyes and therefore spatial perception and the interaction with objects arises through the active correlation of the separate data of touch with the data of vision. In the case of either the blind patient who can later see or the infant who learns about distance, this correlation is not instantaneous but is a long, slow, developmental process. In other words, in the case both of the blind subject who recovers their vision and the infant in their normal process of development, upon opening their eyes the subject does not immediately respond to patterns of light on the retina but, through a more lengthy cognitive process that involves correlating vision and touch, 'learns to see'.

After several hundred years of experimental evidence and surgical operations, should the question not be resolved by now? As Heller states, 'the many studies of the restoration of sight do not provide unequivocal answers to Molyneux's question' (1991: 241). The answer is negative for the following reasons. First, the Molyneux question is a classic example of an attempt to gain privileged access to the content of another person's mental state and cognitive processes, in this case of the blind by the sighted. However sophisticated the questioning, qualitative inquiry is hampered in this respect by the absolute inability to access another person's thought processes, and this problem persists in current examinations of experiences of blindness. There remain only fragments and imaginations. Secondly, there are complexities in the interpretation of the evidence over what counts as 'blindness' and 'sight', and in historical accounts these have not been systematised or standardised. Whether congenital or adventitious, and irrespective of the differing sensitivities to light that form the continuum from sighted to non-sighted, the historical evidence remains difficult to unpick as this information was not identified in the accounts. And thirdly, the post-operative experience varies greatly between patients, so that 'learning how to see' (Gregory and Wallace 1963; Gregory 1967; Sacks 1995) is different according to the plasticity and adaptability of each person, and the level of previous retinal damage.

For example, von Senden in 1932 agreed with Platner's findings, arguing that the tactile experience of the blind is entirely non-spatial, the blind person having no proper spatial representation of the objects touched. 'What are features of shape to us are for him [*sic*] wholly unspatial, purely tactile distinctions of sensation or dynamic movement', he argues; 'they are distinctions in the constancy of sequence and ordering of impressions' (1960: 49). Consequently he concludes that there are no 'absolute spatial concepts' for the blind, and that for the blind person there are only 'relational concepts, ordered sequences and schemata' (1960: 61). This he infers from a selective reading of post-operative accounts. Their descriptions of phenomena while sightless are related primarily to the peripersonal touch-space around the body, making it difficult to conceptualise a shape or figure lying beyond reach of hand or cane. Interviews conducted and published in a weekly newspaper with the congenitally blind subject Joan Getaz, questioned in 1928, fuelled further the public imagination of blind spatial experience. Without prior visual experience she conceptualised a tree serially and schematically as a temporal, textural sequence of trunk, branch, and leaves. Due to confusion over relative sizes compared with the body, Getaz apparently assumed that the tree was not much larger than a man. From this specious observation in the popular press, von Senden concludes that there is a difference between the visual and the tactile fields. The schema or ordered sequence is therefore not a 'real consciousness of space' (von Senden 1960: 69).

This view is not widely held. Recalling Berkeley's dogmatic assertion that our spatial knowledge comes primarily through touch, and that touch informs and appends vision, Warnock (in von Senden 1960: 322) and Jones (1975: 461) regarded von Senden's view, that the congenitally blind have no spatial concepts, as equally dogmatic and unsupported by evidence. A more recent report examining tactile mapping suggests that the congenitally blind 'may encode space in a serial, egocentric manner' (Kitchin et al. 1997: 233), a self-referential, route-type representation of space. This perhaps encapsulates the contemporary spatial imagination by the sighted of the congenitally blind: the assumption of tactuo-spatial 'images' or inner mental representations, especially of the static kind. More recent psychology endeavours to escape these representational models, and from Gibson (1966) and Piaget and Inhelder (1971) onwards they have stressed how spatial perceptions can occur without spatial 'pictures' or inner mental representations, a spatiality resulting from active movement, informed by kinaesthesia (Gibson 1950: 224; Karlsson and Magnusson 1994: 10 n. 1). Indeed, Jones (1975: 466) argues specifically against what he calls the 'visual map' theory, and asserts instead the importance of motor organisation, citing empirical evidence for this. Returning to an insight by Diderot, when first opening our eyes we learn to compare sensations by experience, thereby admitting a *temporal* component to spatial perception. For cross-modal perception to occur for the Molyneux patient or for Diderot, there is a temporal aspect to sensory experience that forges associations between the sense modalities, thereby involving kinaesthesia, the memory of touch-patterns, and other sensory-motor interventions. These observations would entail a modified answer to the Molyneux question, where what is commonly known as 'visuo-spatial working memory' (Baddely 1992) relies on 'mental images' in the blind that are neither specifically visual nor spatial, as Graven observes (2003: 102), and so memory allows the transfer of information between modalities. But at some level there is convergence between the sensory modalities, so that 'a cognitive vision-touch link [is] derived from converging subsystems' (Graven 2003: 108). In terms of the absolute pragmatic experience of working memory, his evidence suggests that memory alone is not the intermediary of cross-modal transfer. Instead, there are underlying encoding processes at a 'lower cognitive level' than memory (2003: 108), encoding experiences from different sensory subsystems. In other words, while memory might allow cross-modal transfer between modalities such as vision and touch, perception is more amodal than cross-modal. Where does this leave the experiences of eyes and hands, of blindness and spatial imagination?

Quite apart from questions of spatial perception, Alberto Valvo (1971) covered what he termed the 're-education' of newly sighted subjects, namely the long rehabilitative process of learning to see and the required adjustments in personality for this to be successful. In his *Sight Restoration after Long-Term Blindness* he reviews some previous case studies, including his own blind subject H.S., and is keen to dispel the illusion that ophthalmic surgery provides an instant solution to blindness: 'Surgical intervention is but the first stage in a long process going far beyond physiological changes to the eye' (Valvo 1971: 3). In fact, Valvo noted the infrequency with which subjects responded positively to the 'gift' of sight, those who effectively renounced their previously tactile world of assurance in favour of a less certain, but more visual, world:

> The congenitally blind person especially, has to face the prospect of a difficult struggle before reaching a stage at which his vision permits him to understand the world around him. For a period of time varying with each patient, these people experience a confusing proliferation of perceptions, and they must learn to see as a child learns to walk. (1971: 4)

As will be shown in the following brief summaries of case studies, few formerly blind subjects respond positively to the introduction of the visual modality, as Maria Theresia von Paradis and the well-known case studies in the psychology literature of S.B. and 'Virgil' poignantly demonstrate. The 'gift' of sight can be transformed into a curse, the newly sighted subject encounters stresses in negotiating this newly visual world, becomes ill and depressed, and their lives can be foreshortened. As von Senden (1960) and Valvo (1971) were both aware, once the initial euphoria in encountering the visual world has faded, the subject in some cases becomes overwhelmed by the huge cognitive burden of becoming a visual being, of continually having to learn to see. As a result, they effectively shut down their own visual world. Valvo identifies a further factor in the onset of depression, the significant personality adjustments required for any blind subject, especially in later life, to renounce the assured tactile world for the challenges of a newly visual world. Such formerly blind subjects had not just built an experiential world around touch, but had also developed a pronounced blind identity that included tactile habits, distinct ways of living, and personality traits. The tasks and movements that were achieved with relative ease as a blind person would become manifestly more difficult as a newly sighted person, and Valvo reports the patient H.S. expressing that 'he was more disabled than before' in the first few weeks after his operation (1971: 30). The process of renouncing their tactile ways of living to accommodate a new visual modality was described unequivocally by one of Valvo's patients: 'I had to die as a blind person to be reborn as a seeing person' (1971: 4).

Conclusion

This chapter has shown that some of the foundational concepts that Gregory and Wallace, Sacks, and others employed in their case studies were premised on records of surgical experiments and philosophical inquiry that were rooted in the later part of the seventeenth century and the beginning of the eighteenth, reaching a critical nexus between Berkeley's adoption of Locke's ideas and Cheselden's report to the Royal Society in 1728. The next chapter will document the popularisation of that critical moment afterwards in France through Voltaire, Condillac, Buffon, and others, when philosophical investigations into perception were married with discussions based on medical evidence from Cheselden, Brisseau, Daviel, and others. An

Enlightenment fascination with blindness and the seeing of 'truth' was maintained, but with more specifically pedagogical implications. Voltaire's celebrated articulation of these ideas, 'We learn to see just as we learn to speak and read' (1991: 68), could be said to form the basis for our understanding of the recovery of sight after blindness ever since Cheselden, and is recognisable within the case studies discussed here. Being able finally to see an object for the first time, yet remaining confused by it, the blind subject correlates the newly visual blobs of colour they see with what was familiar in their previously tactile world. In that case, ocular surgery is not enough. It is only through cross-modal perceptions, active correlations between vision and touch, that the visual system as a whole renders the sensations meaningful. Having touched their objects, two of the case study subjects, Bradford and Virgil, are reported to have resolved the sometimes confusing, chaotic patterns of light and colour into more familiar form. In the encounter with the lathe in the Science Museum, Bradford is reported as saying: 'Now that I've felt it, I can see!' (Gregory and Wallace 1963: 31). Likewise Virgil, having touched a statue of a gorilla at a zoo while simultaneously seeing its visual patterns behind the cage, was, in Sacks's words, a 'spectacular example of how touching could make seeing possible' (1995: 127).

Having summarised some standout ideas from the case studies, a brief coda. As the depression and withdrawal into blindness of certain case studies would suggest, there are intense emotions released in adjusting to a newly visual world. Although there are examples of films that challenge the nature and power of seeing (e.g. Michael Powell's *Peeping Tom*, 1960), there is often a tendency to soften complex psychological truths, to turn emotional journeys into melodrama. Sacks's study of Virgil in *An Anthropologist on Mars* (1995) was adapted into the mawkish Hollywood production *At First Sight* (1999). Sacks had initially prepared for meetings with Virgil by reading Gregory and Wallace's monograph alongside other case studies (Sacks 1995: 103), and so there are intentional commonalities in the portrayal of both post-operative subjects. There remain recognisable tropes and phenomena shared between the case study of S.B. and Virgil as depicted by Sacks and in the film. A further emotional element to these narratives becomes manifest in that sighted subjects sometimes push for ophthalmic surgery on behalf of their blind lovers, and certainly Virgil's partner Amy desired something of him that Valvo had earlier identified, namely a 'renaissance of personality' or 'a completely new personality configuration' (1971: 3) in the shift from blind to sighted subject, tactile to visual perception.

Brian Friel's play *Molly Sweeney* works as a series of monologues that deal unmelodramatically with the emotional fallout of a compound case of the recovery of sight after blindness, based heavily on Virgil (see Feeney 2007). Certain phrases that occur throughout the material covered in this chapter, from Voltaire ('We learn to see, exactly as we learn to speak and read') to Valvo ('a renaissance of personality'), from Gregory ('learning to see') to Sacks (Virgil 'found himself between two worlds, at home in neither'), become voiced through the characters, the eponymous blind subject Molly, her sighted husband Frank who wishes for a miraculous recovery, and the doctor who performs the operation. Since several of the case studies faced post-operative vision at a later stage in their lives, with Valvo (1971) we identified a pattern of reversion to a previously blind way of living, a withdrawal from the sighted world that indicated clinical depression. Friel's play is based on an understanding of these case studies, voicing different hopes and emotions through the perspectives of blind subject, sighted lover, and ophthalmic surgeon. At one point, Molly nostalgically reflects on a time before her vision was restored by the operation, and takes pleasure in remembering her previously tactile world of sensuous envelopment without visual distractions. Reminding herself, and indeed the audience, of the active undergoing of corporeal sensation which is part of everyday embodied experience for both blind and sighted alike, we leave Molly with the last words. The case studies were perhaps justifiably fascinated by the unfolding complex emotional arc of disappointment and depression after sight restoration. But in one of her monologues, the fictional Molly vocalises something unambiguously positive about the pleasures of her previously tactile world:

> And how could I have told those other doctors how much pleasure my world offered me? From my work, from the radio, from walking, from music, from cycling. But especially from swimming. Oh I can't tell you the joy I got from swimming. I used to think – and I know this sounds silly – but I really did believe I got more pleasure, more delight, than sighted people can ever get. Just offering yourself to the experience – every pore open and eager for that world of pure sensation, of sensation alone – that could not have been enhanced by sight – experience that existed only by touch and feel; and moving swiftly and rhythmically through that enfolding world; and the sense of such assurance, such liberation, such concordance with it. (Friel 1994: 24)

Chapter 4

Voltaire, Buffon, and Blindness in France

The validation of sensation

If, after Descartes, the issues raised around blindness for Locke and Berkeley originate in philosophical inquiry and speculative epistemology, then the results of surgical intervention lie within scientific experimentation. Locke's empiricism was taken up in Europe as a challenge to the entrenched rationalism of Descartes, and a new emphasis on the centrality of experience and sensation was kickstarted by Voltaire in exile, and developed into a fully fledged sensationism through Condillac. It is some measure of the 'fruitfulness' of the Molyneux question, thinks Ernst Cassirer in his monumental study *The Philosophy of the Enlightenment*, that it continued to stimulate responses in France several decades later. Voltaire in his *Éléments de la philosophie de Newton* offered 'an extensive exposition of the problem', and Condillac apparently declared that 'it contains the source and key to all modern psychology' (Cassirer 1979: 109). Cheselden's 1728 report to the Royal Society in London provided further stimulus to the French intellectual imagination. After Voltaire introduced a French readership to Cheselden's case study through the *Elements*, in successive years there followed further discussion of the role of the senses in the production of knowledge, including Condillac's *Essai sur l'origine des connaissances humaines* ['An essay on the origin of human knowledge'] (1746) and, in a revised form, *Traité des sensations* ['Treatise on the sensations'] (1754); Diderot's *Lettre sur les aveugles à l'usage de ceux qui voient* ['Letter on the blind for the use of those who see'] (1749); and George Buffon's *Histoire naturelle, générale et particulière* ['Natural history of man'] (1749). A chapter in La Mettrie's *Histoire naturelle de l'âme* ['Natural history of the soul'] (1745) was entitled 'Stories that confirm that all ideas come from the senses', simultaneously invoking the familiar Peripatetic axiom while reaffirming the centrality of sensation in epistemological inquiry. In the wake of new scientific and surgical discoveries, French commentators such as the sensationists often considered the fact that sensations had a source outside the body to be an emotional matter, but also that there was no substantial separation between the emotional and the cognitive aspects (Riskin 2002: 49). After Cheselden, sensation and sensationism in France were going to take a radical new trajectory.

What was it in the wake of Molyneux's question and Cheselden's surgery that so piqued the French imagination, that Condillac regarded as so foundational to the beginnings of psychology? H. W. Carr, in his preface to an English translation of Condillac's *Traité*, surmises: 'In Condillac's day philosophic speculation was concentrated on the problem of the nature of the dependence of knowledge on the functioning of the various special sense organs. It was primarily a psychological rather than a metaphysical problem' (Condillac 1930: xvi). Likewise, Cassirer characterises this period as lying between epistemology and psychology, as attention was being drawn away from purely optical mechanisms of perception, outlined so clearly in Descartes' *Dioptrique* for example, and increasingly towards the role of the faculty of judgement in any act of perception. Later this led to the psychological physiology of Pierre Cabanis, whose doctrine of *sensibilité organique* [organic sensibility] in *Rapports du physique et du moral de l'homme* (1802) considered all intellectual processes to derive from 'sensibility', a property of the nervous system.

The root of this uptake for Voltaire, Diderot, and Cabanis was the striking originality of Locke's *Essay Concerning Human Understanding*. The fourth edition was translated into French in 1700 by Pierre Coste, not only popularising a new brand of radical empiricism for a European audience, but also widening awareness of, and speculation upon, the Molyneux question. In 1709, the same year as *The Tatler* reported the cataract operation of Grant the oculist, the Frenchman Michel Brisseau published his *Traité de la cataracte et du glaucome* ['Treatise on cataracts and glaucoma'] based on recent anatomical confirmations of the location of the cataract in the crystalline lens. This essay offered technical recommendations for ophthalmic procedures that went beyond the prior 'couching' techniques of barber-surgeons, which proved controversial in the medical community. It would be five years after Brisseau's death in 1743 before the technique for the extraction of the lens known as extracapsular cataract extraction would be refined, performed, and published by Jacques Daviel in his *Lettre sur les maladies des yeux* ['Letter on the diseases of the eye']

(1748), along with a detailed report to the French Royal Academy, 'Sur une nouvelle méthode de guérir la cataracte par l'extraction du crystallin' ['A new method of curing cataracts by extraction of the lens'] (1754). Daviel's extraction technique, supposedly performed in 206 operations of which 182 were successful, increased the success rate from more primitive couching methods, and a variant is still used today (Jampel 1998; Diderot suggests that there were 226 operations, 1916b: 144 n. 1). Although no direct philosophical interest was shown in Brisseau's discovery at the time, Denis Diderot's *Additions á la lettre sur les aveugles* ['Addition to the preceding letter'], written around thirty-four years later and appended to his famous *Lettre*, refers to Daviel's great surgical reputation and goes into some detail about one of his patients.

Even in the more relaxed circumstances of the Regency period after the death of Louis XIV, Voltaire attracted trouble by writing verses critical of the Regent, Philippe, Duke of Orléans, which led to his imprisonment in the Bastille without trial (Albert 1997). Nine years later, arrested this time for quarrelling in public with a nobleman, Voltaire feared returning to prison, so he volunteered self-imposed exile in England in 1726, which was granted. What began as a self-inflicted punishment shifted gradually into anglophilia, as he mingled with famous English novelists and playwrights of the age, and was most impressed with the satirist Jonathan Swift. His *Letters Concerning the English Nation* (1733), subsequently published in French as *Lettres philosophiques* (1734), was based on this three-year exposure to literary England, with its comparative religious tolerance and free intercourse of ideas. The book failed to impress the French public, and so on returning to France he turned instead to English philosophy and science, specifically Locke and Newton. Some measure of the esteem and influence that Locke enjoyed in Britain and abroad is evident in the *Lettres*, where he writes of Locke: 'So many philosophers having written the romance of the soul, a sage has arrived who has modestly written its history. Locke has set forth human reason just as an excellent anatomist explains the parts of the human body' (in Cassirer 1979: 94).

Voltaire's continued fascination with British intellectual life led to the popularisation in France of Newton's ideas, with their questions of geometry, optics, and perspective, and this found expression in his *Elements de la philosophie de Newton* (1738), published the same year in translation as *Elements of Newton's Philosophy*. It 'was a stimulus of the greatest importance to new thought in France' (Morley 1878: 54). Despite its title, the work ranged widely, encompassing not only Newton's writing on optics but also summarising sections of Locke's *Essay* and Berkeley's *Theory of Vision*, the better to support arguments on the perception of objects at a distance. In order for Voltaire to illustrate these ideas for non-specialist readers, he inevitably included discussion of the restoration of sight in Cheselden's patient, and the necessity of transfer between sense modalities in the acquisition of perspective. Likewise, Buffon's fourth volume of his monumental *Histoire naturelle*, written between 1749 and 1788 and published in thirty-six volumes, dealt with the senses, and one chapter, 'On the sense of seeing', directly revisited Cheselden's patient in order to argue strongly that all vision is corrected through the sense of touch, so that 'we may consider sight as a species of touching, though very different from what we commonly understand by that sense' (1797: 152). What Buffon means by this particular form of touching and its relation to vision will be examined in the final section.

'We learn to see just as we learn to speak and read': Voltaire

Voltaire's *Dictionnaire philosophique* (1764) was written towards the end of his life and provides a useful snapshot of his erudite style and restless inquiry. It consists of a series of substantial summaries of key ideas, succinct but substantial statements that summarise knowledge in that area. His entry on 'Imagination' touches upon blindness and the role of sight for furnishing the imagination of an individual. Several decades earlier, Joseph Addison had written a series of twelve articles 'On the pleasures of the imagination' for the literary periodical he co-founded in 1712, *The Spectator*. In these essays and a book from 1699 detailing his Grand Tour of Europe, the idea of the 'sublime' took root, to be developed further by Edmund Burke. But it was the philosophical content of the idea of the imagination that excited Voltaire. He states approvingly that the first of Addison's essays starts with the generalisation that 'the sense of sight is the only one which furnishes the imagination with ideas' (Voltaire 1884: 158), but this is a mistranslation. In actuality, Addison starts the essay series with a useful comparison between the senses of sight and touch in the perception of distance, consistent with Locke's argument about the place of inference and reflection in seeing: 'Our Sight is the most perfect and most delightful of all our Senses. It fills the Mind with the largest Variety of Ideas, converses with its Objects at the greatest Distance, and continues the longest in Action without being tired or satiated with its proper Enjoyments' (1712: 137). Nevertheless, Voltaire's response in the essay 'Imagination' was to petition for the role of the other senses:

> A man born blind still hears, in his imagination, the harmony which no longer vibrates upon his ear; he still continues listening as in a trance or dream; the objects which have resisted or yielded to his hands produce a similar effect in his head or mind. It is true that the sense of sight alone supplies images; and as it is a kind of touching or feeling which extends even to the distance of the stars, its immense diffusion enriches the imagination more than all the other senses put together. (1884: 158–9)

While this is a characteristically poetic articulation of what the imagination might mean for both the sighted and the blind, it is unclear how qualified Voltaire was to assert this. By attempting to claim knowledge and speak on behalf of the blind, is this anything other than the well-worn trope of a sighted imaginary of the non-sighted other, donning the 'cloak' of blindness as Descartes had done to speculate on epistemological matters? By examining Voltaire's writing on blindness elsewhere, especially a crucial section of an earlier text of popular science, we are in a stronger position to answer.

If, after his exile from France, Voltaire failed to inspire enthusiasm for English literature in the French public in *Lettres philosophiques*, a shift to more practically minded science in his *Éléments de la philosophie de Newton* was notably more successful. Given its title, a reader of Voltaire's *Éléments* might wonder why such an 'extended exposition' of Molyneux's problem was necessary among appraisals of the titular scientist's celebrated discoveries in optics and physics. The answer lies in Voltaire's faithfulness to the British empiricists and a challenge to the entrenched Cartesianism of the scientists in France. Vision, as Voltaire learns from Locke and especially Berkeley, is simply not reducible to the mechanisms of optics. For example, in Chapter VI, entitled 'In what manner we know distances, magnitudes, figures, and situations', Voltaire summarises Berkeley's position that our perceptions of an object's qualities, such as shape (Figure), size (Magnitude), and distance from the observer, 'are not sensations but inferences', are not 'the immediate revelations of sight, but the products of association and intellectual construction', and are 'not directly judged by vision, but by imagination and experience' (Morley 1878: 54). Emphasising the role of judgement and custom in vision is consistent with Locke's and Berkeley's explanations. However, Voltaire's expositions in *Éléments* stay firmly within the confines of the British philosophers' systems, and his mission to popularise the new philosophical contributions was restricted to explanation rather than sustained critical engagement. Later, Condillac would take a more critical position and advance a distinct argument concerning language and the senses in his *Traité*, to which we return below.

Initially it would seem rather arbitrary that the *Éléments* contains Voltaire's most extensive discussion of blindness. In the text Voltaire summarises some important epistemological steps from Locke and Berkeley concerning the perception of objects, perspective, and therefore the relationship between vision and touch that are now familiar to us. After invoking the Molyneux question, Voltaire offers a concise appraisal of the kind of empirical evidence that might answer it, namely Cheselden's removal of cataracts in 1728. As we know, there remains a central epistemological problem within any theory that validates the input of sensation as the pre-eminent building block for more complex ideas, including imagination and recollection. But Voltaire has reason to break from mechanistic models of optics in explanations of visual perception, and is explicitly aware that angles, shapes, and patterns of light falling upon the retina do not in themselves provide information of size, distance, or shape of external objects, due to other contextual qualities such as different lighting conditions or prior familiarity with that object. This is how Cassirer puts the central problematic:

> In the midst of phenomena which are immediately perceived by our senses, and which we cannot avoid, something has been discovered which lies beyond all the limits of perception. The distance between objects appears by its very nature to be imperceptible. And yet it is an element which is absolutely essential to the structure of our conception of the world. *The spatial form of perceptions is fused with its sense material*; and yet it is not given in the material alone, nor can it be analytically reduced to this material. Thus the form of perceptions constitutes a foreign body in the only accessible world of immediate sense data which cannot be eliminated without causing this world to collapse. (1979: 111, emphasis added)

A pithy sentence by Berkeley illustrates this point well: 'distance is in its own nature imperceptible and yet it is perceived by sight' (*Vision* §11). The previous chapter showed how he resolved this by expanding the basic concept of perception to mean something beyond mere sensation, to include the activity of representation. Consequently, the spatial component of an object does not lie within a particular perception, and belongs neither to vision not to touch alone, but is present within the play of sense-impressions and prior associations. As Cassirer explains: 'The idea of space is not, therefore, strictly speaking an element of sense consciousness but an expression of a process which goes on in consciousness' (1979: 112). Berkeley's contribution was not just a response to Locke in England, then, but was also adapted by leading figures in France, including Voltaire, Condillac, and Diderot, who modify certain details but accept that 'visual impressions in themselves include a certain "spatiality"' (Cassirer 1979: 113).

Voltaire illustrates this point about the spatiality of the senses by turning to that familiar hypothetical figure, 'some Person born blind' (1991: 63). In among the now familiar details, however, is this refreshingly modern observation, the first sentence of which would be echoed most effectively over two hundred years later in a report by psychologist Richard Gregory (Gregory and Wallace 1963):

> We learn to see just as we learn to speak and read. [...] The sudden and almost uniform Judgments, which every Mind forms at a certain Age of Distances, Magnitudes, and Situations, make us think it only necessary to open the Eyes, in order to see Things as they are. But this is a Mistake; the Aid of the other Senses is essential to this Effect. (1991: 68–9)

Opening the eyes is not enough to see, and therefore vision consists of other processes and relies on other sensory input in order to discern qualities such as size, shape, and distance. This is the significant conclusion of Locke and Berkeley's theory of vision. But Voltaire re-describes these theories not only to perform the work of the popularisation of ideas unfamiliar or alien to a French readership, but to shake up the entrenched Cartesianism of his native land by directly contesting some well-known tenets of Descartes' doubt concerning the senses, notably the unreliability of the senses in the path to true knowledge, especially in Part IV of *Discourse on Method* and section 31 of *Meditations on First Philosophy*. With the seeds of sensory doubt sown so extensively for Descartes, the contrary position of Voltaire's articulation of Locke has increased resonance:

> We are therefore very much in the wrong when we say our Senses deceive us. Each of them discharge the Function for which Nature intended them. They assist each other mutually, in conveying to the Soul by Means of Experience, such a Measure of Knowledge as our

Condition admits. We demand of our Senses, what they were not formed to bestow. We are for knowing from our Eyes Solidity, Magnitude, Distance &c. but the Touch must unite in this with the Sight, and Experience with both. (1991: 70–1)

In order for Voltaire to argue this, he must walk the reader through highlights of Locke's and Berkeley's ideas about vision, while being aware of Descartes' examples in the *Meditations*. At one stage Voltaire gives the same brief example of walking up to a stone tower that appears circular from afar, but on approach and through touching reveals itself as 'quadrangular'. The example serves opposing ends, however, for Descartes' example (*Meditation* VI) built up evidence against the reliability of the senses, whereas Voltaire wishes to establish the utility of association between the senses in building up a more robust and evidence-based picture of the world. 'The measurable and tangible Object therefore is one Thing, and the Object of Vision another', he states (1991: 61). Cassirer (1979) would see in this the tendency in subsequent philosophy and psychology to assume incommensurate sensory worlds, where the space of sight and that of touch are considered entirely separate and experimented on accordingly. We will return to this shortly, but an argument about size constancy veers directly into the territory of blindness and Cheselden's surgery to restore vision.

As his departure point, and against previous classical scholarship, Berkeley in his *Essay* proposed that the spatial properties of objects did not reside in the objects themselves, but rather that distance is perceived through experience. In section §53 he argued for a form of size constancy, that is, the same cues that evoke distance also evoke size, and so we do not first perceive size and then calculate distance. Quite reasonably, Voltaire echoes this argument for size constancy, arguing that if we see a person at a distance of four feet they still appear the same size as when they are eight feet away, even if the angle subtended through the lens upon the retina is much greater in the former case than the latter. 'Whence is it, that my Perception contradicts the Mechanism of my Organs in this Manner?' he asks (1991: 62). For clearly the explanation of the size and distance of perceived objects lies not in the geometry of lines and angles in themselves, but through prolonged experience and correlations between vision and touch built up over time. The centrality of such experiences over time is what allows the cognitive processing ('Perception') of sensory data ('the Mechanism of my Organs'), and size constancy and the sense of depth perspective that pertained to Voltaire's and

Descartes' earlier erroneous perceptions, later corrected through updated sensory information, of square towers appearing circular from afar. We might add here a category of visual illusions such as mirages, or Descartes' straightforward example of the refraction of light through water which makes a stick appear bent, discussed in the reply to point 9 of the Sixth Objection to the *Meditations* (2008: 437–9) and, earlier, the first discourse of *Dioptrique* (1965: 67–8). Descartes' reply to an objection about validating a visual illusion of the stick by correlating it with the kind of tactile experience familiar from childhood is apparently 'not [...] sufficient to correct the visual error' because this is another form of sensation, and by implication potentially erroneous, and so 'only the intellect can correct the errors of the senses' (Descartes 2008: 439). To argue against such rigidly Cartesian innate principles that validate the intellect over sensory experience, therefore, Voltaire elucidates his point for the reader about the centrality of experience by considering the example of 'some Person born blind, and restored to the Sense of Sight' (1991: 63), namely Cheselden's patient.

Voltaire's justification for turning to the example of blindness lies in his earlier assertion, based in turn on Berkeley, that qualities of shape (Figure), size (Magnitude), and distance from the observer are not present in the visual perception of an object by itself, and that prolonged experience and associations between the senses need to take place over time. One test for this, thinks Voltaire, is to consider a person suddenly able to see for the first time. If they are able to discern those physical and dimensional qualities of an object simply through the patterns of light on the retina, then this categorically opposes both Locke's initial answer to the Molyneux question and Berkeley's more developed theory of vision, wherein prolonged experience and prior exposure through the senses is necessary. Voltaire reasons: 'For if this blind Person, at the Moment he received Sight, had judged of Distances, Magnitudes and Situations, it had been true that the optick Angles, formed that instant in his *Retina*, had been the immediate Causes of his Thoughts' (1991: 63, original italics). The only way to settle this issue definitively, then, is to examine an actual case study. Cheselden is described by Voltaire as 'one of those famous Surgeons, who unite a great Extent of Knowledge with Dexterity in Operations' (1991: 64). There is, however, no evidence that Voltaire knew Cheselden, and his writing style in general often involves a patchwork of highly embellished or exaggerated descriptions and observations for the benefit of the general reader. In discussing the patient prior to the operation, for example, Voltaire seems astonished by his 'indifference' towards his sightless condition, and with an incredulous tone Voltaire reports: 'He could not very well conceive, that the Sense of Sight would contribute much to his Happiness' (1991: 64). This is probably a rhetorical strategy for the sighted reader.

The results of Cheselden's operation were covered extensively earlier, but Voltaire's version of the events highlights a few noteworthy differences and exaggerations. Observation of Cheselden's patient immediately after the operation, according to Voltaire, did indeed confirm Locke and Berkeley's position, that the recognition of objects and their qualities is not instantaneous. 'For a long Time he distinguished neither Magnitude, Distance, Situation, nor even Figure', Voltaire declares, before elaborating:

> An object of an Inch placed before his Eyes, that concealed an House from his Sight, appeared to him as big as the House. Every Thing he saw, seemed at first to be upon his Eyes, and to touch them, as the Objects of the Sense of Feeling touch the Skin. He could not distinguish what he had judged round, by the Help of his Hands, from what he had judged square; nor discern with his Eyes, whether what his Hands had perceived to be above or below, were really above or below. (1991: 64–5)

Unsurprisingly, the results are unequivocal, with Voltaire providing a summary of Locke and Berkeley's ideas along with a somewhat embellished transcription of Cheselden's report. The episode in the surgeon's report to the Royal Society dealing with the patient's perception of a two-dimensional painting now became transcribed into the language of heightened wonder and sensationalism:

> He could not perceive, till after two Months Experience, that Pictures only represented solid Bodies, and when, after so long a Trial of his new Sense [Cheselden's 1728 report says several months], he had thought, that Bodies, and not Surfaces only, were in the painted Tables, he put his Hand to them, and was amazed that he did not feel those solid Bodies, of which he began to perceive the Representations. He asked which of the Senses deceived him, that of Feeling, or that of Seeing. (1991: 65)

Clearly, it is not simply patterns of light on the retina that allow the visual perception of three-dimensional objects, whether they are cubes and spheres or tables and painted representations of tables. Patterns of light on the retina, or as Voltaire persists in putting it,

'Angles formed in our Eyes', are 'of no Manner of Use to him without the Aid of Experience, and the other Senses' (1991: 66).

In the later *Dictionnaire philosophique* of 1764, Voltaire's essay on 'Distance' mentions angles, the geometry of light, and the necessity of experience in remarkably similar terms, and some passages from the *Éléments* are reproduced verbatim in the *Dictionnaire*. Here the problem of how one conceives of the idea of distance is put to the reader, and we are guided through the reasoning process. If we are able to gauge the hardness or softness of an object directly through touch, or judge something either bitter or sweet through taste, there is no immediate way to judge distance, and so this is achieved 'by means of an intermediate idea' (Voltaire 1904: 135). If the concept of distance cannot be extrapolated directly through the sense of touch or audition, then it is equally not to be derived from the mechanics of vision, the calculations of angles of light through the gelatinous humour of the eye, Voltaire argues. Again, as in the *Éléments*, he invokes the example of a blind man with restored vision: 'For if this blind man, the moment that he opens his eyes, can correctly judge of distances, dimensions and situations, it would be true that the optical angles suddenly formed in his retina were the immediate cause of his decisions' (1904: 138). Moreover, although much of his earlier material reappears almost verbatim here, one section dealing with his relationship to Cheselden stands out. He portrays himself in the third person as the 'author of the "Elements of Newton", who had seen a great deal of Cheselden', whereas in actuality no previous mention of meeting Cheselden occurs, even in the *Éléments*. Perhaps this was an attempt to retrospectively impose the force of his personality on to historical events, further blurring the line between historical event and fictional embellishment. Nevertheless, Voltaire states here that, after the operation in 1728, '[t]he adventure of the man born blind was known in France towards the year 1735' (1904: 140), and it is clear that the limitations of methodology and the lack of systematic note-taking, evident within Cheselden's own report to the Royal Society, is a frustration for Voltaire. Likewise, with a later cataract operation in Paris (presumably Daviel's), rigorous observation is lacking and the findings are frustratingly forever lost to posterity:

> And even when the same operation of the cataract was performed in Paris on a young man who was said to have been deprived of sight from his cradle, the operators neglected to attend to the daily development of the sense of sight in him and to the progress of nature. The fruit of this operation was therefore lost to philosophy. (1904: 140)

This is a telling deviation from the earlier text, for if Voltaire's purpose here is predominantly a rearticulation of elements of Locke and Berkeley's arguments, with the vindication of Locke's initial negative answer to the Molyneux question, this passage hints at the potential for a more refined position on the matter in terms of the psychology of his intimation elsewhere that we 'learn how to see'. Unfortunately this impulse remains unexamined, and both texts unexpectedly veer into more fanciful territory, extending the role of experience in visual perception into a kind of grammar.

Later Voltaire returns to firmer ground by considering another everyday example within the sighted world, that of noticing a distant human figure on a rooftop. Bringing in his earlier arguments about size constancy he now offers an explanation as to why, at a distance, the ambiguity of the figure is resolved when, on approaching more closely, in actuality the figure is revealed not to be two feet high and a sculpture, but a full-sized human. Combined with the insights gained from considering Cheselden's patient and the resolution of the Molyneux problem, we now come full circle in this section, for this is the justification for the declaration about learning to see:

> From all this we must absolutely conclude, that Distances, Magnitudes, and Situations, are not, properly speaking, Things to be seen, that is to say, the proper and immediate Objects of Sight. The proper and immediate Object of Sight is nothing in Nature but coloured Light; all the rest we only attain to know by Length of Time and Experience. We learn to see, exactly as we learn to speak and read. (1991: 68)

And in this process of learning to see we depend on the experience of other senses, as we would otherwise have no practical means for discerning 'Extent, Length, Breadth, and Depth' of objects (1991: 69). Thus it is that imperceptible things, like the distance between an object and ourselves, or perspective based on occlusion, come to be seen by a sighted subject over time.

Language, gesture, and the sensation: Condillac and Diderot

Within the *Éléments* Voltaire had briefly written on language and signs. The seeds of an argument concerning the role of the senses in the origin of language, the association between sign and sensation, and the circulation of those signs would develop and come to fruition for his countrymen Diderot and Buffon a decade later, but it was not novel. A sign theory of perception, in which sensory experiences are arbitrary signs (like words) for external objects and properties, was present in Descartes, and would reappear with Helmholtz. But it is worth briefly highlighting how Voltaire's generic argument about signs and the senses shifts for Diderot into a more sophisticated and specific argument concerning the blind and the possibility of a tactile language in *Lettre sur les aveugles*, but also the possibilities for a language of gesture for the deaf and the deaf-mute in the later *Lettre sur les sourds et muets* (1751). Essentially this thread between the two works starts with Voltaire's observation concerning the connection, but also slippage, between the sensory impressions of an object, the abstraction involved in the idea of that object, and the inscriptions as signs that are employed to evoke such an object in its absence. Voltaire argues that there is an 'annexing' of the association between something seen, say a gold coin, with the abstracted idea of 'yellow', or when we hear a word enunciated: 'we cannot help annexing the Idea of that Coin to the Sound we hear uttered' (1991: 69). This is an arbitrary connection which relies on sensory association, but from which an elementary linguistic theory can be discerned in germinal form. Voltaire explains his concern thus:

> If all Men spoke the same Language, we should always be ready to believe, that there would be a necessary Connection between Words and Ideas. Now in this Point all Men have the same Language, with Respect to Imagination. Nature tells it to all that when you have seen Colours for a certain Time, your Imagination will represent to you, in the same Manner, all the Bodies, in sudden and involuntary Judgment, which you shall form, shall be useful to you during the Course of your Lives. (1991: 69–70)

Although this fragment of argument concerning language is left underdeveloped, the same associative logic is present in the judgement of size, shape, and distance, says Voltaire, through this 'annexing' or an unreflecting, automatic perception that saves us from working out the qualities of objects through geometric inferences about angle, or quality of light through the retina, and so on. We might infer that a similar trope or idea of annexing is present not only in language acquisition, where we seem to automatically make associations between sensory impressions and abstract ideas, but also in perception. The earlier phrase from Voltaire, 'We learn to see just as we learn to speak and read' (1991: 68), is meant here in the most literal way, suggesting an analogue between the psychological functions or mental operations involved in language acquisition and those of visual perception, a neonate or a man born blind learning to see.

Voltaire's fervent belief in the role of sensation and experience above all else was a factor in the rise of what Jay called 'the more uncompromising sensationalism that gained ascendency in the late Enlightenment' (1994: 85). On the one hand, sensationism led to fascinating thought experiments about the role of the senses in the origin of human consciousness. These were played out for example through Diderot's thought experiment in *Lettre sur les sourds et muets*, where a hypothetical man is divided into five, with each part allotted the characteristics of one of the five senses, and Condillac's statue in *Traité des sensations*, which comes slowly to life and becomes animated through successive layers of sensory experience (see Paterson 2007: 48ff.). On the other hand, sensationism becomes somewhat tempered by a residual Cartesian attitude towards vision (the 'noblest of the senses') in France, evident in figures such as Charles de Secondat and Baron de Montesquieu. Another French populariser of learning in philosophy and the sciences, Denis Diderot, was one of the co-founders of that illustrious Enlightenment project, the lavishly illustrated multi-volume survey of the most significant ideas and learning of the time, the original *Encyclopédie*, published between 1751 and 1765. It so happens that Diderot and Voltaire shared a correspondence for twenty-nine years, though they met only on Voltaire's final triumphant return to Paris in 1778, by which time Diderot was an old man. Two of these letters concerned blindness following an exchange of books, Diderot having sent Voltaire his celebrated *Lettre sur les aveugles*, and Voltaire having sent his *Éléments de la philosophie de Newton* in return.

In the *Lettre sur les sourds et muets* there is what Diderot terms a 'muet de convention', translated as 'theoretical mute' (Diderot 1916a: 163). Like the hypothetical blind man, this is another figure of 'les premieres hommes', the first unsocialised men of nature so prevalent at the time through Rousseau and the story of Victor of Aveyron from around 1797. Unlike Rousseau or Condillac, however, Diderot's motivation in outlining a theoretical mute lies not in returning man to a mythical or prelapsarian 'nature'. Nor is he attempting to answer purely epistemological questions, as the hypothetical blind man does. Rather, the *muet de convention* involves a more social inquiry, and as Brewer explains, 'represents a common Enlightenment strategy of presenting and interrogating a figure standing for a supposedly natural or original order so as to establish a critical perspective onto various institutional orders, be they linguistic or social' (2006: 110). However, with an increased focus on sensation and its role in thought experiments concerning vision, memory, and language for Voltaire and, as we shall see, metaphysics for Diderot, three years later Condillac posits a comparable thought experiment involving another blank figure. This was the marble statue that gradually comes to life, involving the successive addition of experience from each of the sense organs. Known as 'Condillac's statue' in the *Traité des sensations*, this was effectively a device to analyse what ideas and faculties we owe to which sense organs, and consequently the role of sensations in the formation of knowledge. The resemblance of Diderot's *muet de convention* as a blank figure and Condillac's statue successively coming to life was sufficiently observed and commented upon that Condillac wrote a pamphlet defending himself from the charge of plagiarism in which, according to Morley, Condillac asserted that 'the Statue was suggested to him by a Mademoiselle Ferrand' (1878: 71). Nevertheless, some cross-pollination of ideas and hypothetical positions would be inevitable given the fact that Condillac introduced Diderot to Rousseau, and Rousseau in his *Confessions* (1770, published 1782) mentions that all three often dined together in Paris at the Hôtel du Panier Fleuri.

Like Voltaire's effort in his *Éléments*, Condillac's *Essai sur l'origin de connaissance humaine* (1746), which preceded his *Traité*, was another straightforward and uncritical attempt to render aspects of Locke's philosophy of perception to a French readership, pressing home the necessity of arguing against Cartesianism that the ultimate source of our ideas lay in impressions made upon the senses, shaped and combined by reflection. Condillac's *Traité* did indeed argue beyond Locke, and Part III of the work, entitled 'How touch teaches the other senses to judge external objects', returns to the Molyneux question in order to extend his argument in the previous section about the role of touch alone and, with a nod to Berkeley, the necessity of touch in perceiving objects in the external world. As Roger Smith argues in his history of the human sciences: 'This analysis made clear the key role that he and others attributed to touch in the acquisition of knowledge of self and non-self and of spatial notions subsequently associated with vision' (1997: 236). While it might seem coldly mechanical, a thought experiment akin to La Mettrie's contemporaneous *L'Homme machine* (1748) that sought rational and reductive explanation for complex physiological and affective processes, here the statue figure demonstrates how the mind gains the capacity to *reflect* upon its sensations at one remove, like Hooke's viewer in his 'perspective box', rather than just passively receiving sensations of various kinds. Condillac's *Essai* puts it this way: 'This manner of successively applying our attention of ourselves to different objects, or to the different parts of one object only, is what we call to *reflect*. Thus we sensibly perceive in what manner reflexion arises from imagination and memory' (in Smith 1997: 236). The emphasis on an abstracted capacity of reflection thereby neatly illustrates a developmental model of transfer across sense modalities whereby the statue becomes aware of space and perspective not merely through optical mechanisms, but only after correlating with other sensory information, primarily, touch. Touch, argues Condillac, is crucial. For it is only in initially touching itself that the statue has a sense of itself, and through touching another neighbouring or contiguous 'foreign body' which does not result in sensation (*Essai* II.v.5), that a concept of external independent objects in space is deducible. The culmination of Condillac's thought experiment is to reject Locke's earlier distinction between 'sensation' and 'reflection', and instead to maintain that 'judgement, reflection, desires, passion and so forth, are only sensation itself differently transformed' (Condillac 1982: 171).

We need not provide a detailed exposition and critique of Condillac's shifting philosophical views on sensation at this stage, but merely note how Condillac shared Locke's tenets and starting point among his countrymen, yet ended up in a distinct position. In the *Traité* he modified his earlier views from the *Essai*, and the purpose of guiding the reader through the thought experiment of an inanimate statue progressively coming to life was to demonstrate what other philosophers had stated, and Voltaire had repeated, namely that 'all our cognitions have been derived from the senses' (*Traité* I.xi.1). In the way that Diderot's blind man of Puiseaux, with a lifetime of tactile experience, has difficulty conceptualising vision in any terms other than touch, the same problem befalls a statue whose first sense is sight, unsupported by any other modalities: 'But how can sight learn from touch? Sight which judges distances it can never reach! Sight which embraces in a moment objects which touch only passes slowly over and never grasps as a whole!' (*Traité* I.xi.1). Shortly afterwards Condillac briefly repeats the genealogy of the thought process, the separation of tactile space from the space of sight in a statue now able to see but unable to experience any other sensations, reversing the order of Molyneux's blind man who touches first, then sees:

> We must credit Mr. Molyneux with being the first to make conjectures on this subject [...] Locke agreed with him that a man born blind whose eyes in later life should be opened to the light would not

be able to distinguish a globe from a cube. This conjecture has since been confirmed by the experiments of Cheselden, which provided the occasion. It seems to me that we are now able to separate with some precision what is due to sight and what is due to touch. (*Traité* I.xi.1)

The contribution of Condillac to the analysis of sensation and the five senses makes him a *philosophe* in the spirit of Diderot, but Condillac's analysis of language and its relation to sensation is more developed, being 'an analysis that treated words as signs for ideas derived from sensation and hence regarded language as a sign system for the representation of knowledge' (Smith 1997: 235). Indeed, a more complete attempt at understanding how knowledge is acquired, including the beginnings of a theory of gesture and non-verbal meaning, occurs in the last book published in his lifetime, *Logic* (1780). Since knowledge ultimately derived from sensory experience, and since words signify the ideas corresponding to the original elements of that experience, the progress of science depends on clarity and order in language. Condillac declares 'that the art of reasoning, reduced to its simplest form can only be a well-formed language' (1982: 410). His position along with Locke that words consist of a conventional, that is, arbitrary and not necessary, system of significations for ideas has been revisited continually, and most famously at the end of the nineteenth century as a basic tenet of modern linguistics through Ferdinand de Saussure. But earlier attempts to consider the relationship between sensation and language, of the inadequacies of articulation, and the necessity of sensory translation across modalities would become crucial for Diderot's suggestion of a tactile language that combines systematic movements and touch as a communication tool, and its eventual development and universal adoption.

Condillac's declaration in the *Traité* that 'judgement, reflection, desires, passion and so forth, are only sensation itself differently transformed' (1982: 171) becomes a definitive statement for a distinct European philosophy made possible only after Locke's positing of the centrality of experience, furthered by Condillac's later writing on sensation and language, which came to be known variously as 'sensationism' [*sensationnisme*] or 'sensationalism' [*sensualisme*] (see e.g. O'Neill 1996). For in parallel with Locke's empiricism, Condillac developed a Gallic correlate to Locke in England, and Herder in Germany, which came to be known by this term. Smith rejects such labelling of Condillac, as the attribution of all mental activity to sensations is rather reductive, whereas Condillac believed that his animated statue did indeed possess an *animus*, a soul. 'Sensation, he wanted to say, enables the faculties to grow in the soul' (Smith 1997: 236). While sensationism developed a bad reputation among Romantic critics who considered this a model of mental passivity, the nature of sensation, the role of movement, and the argument about reflection suggests a more dynamic relationship applicable to active learning in developmental models. Furthermore, we might place such thought experiments within the wider project of a geographically dispersed series of contemporaneous thinkers identified by Goldstein who are 'bringing the psyche into scientific focus', the beginnings of inquiry into cognitive and affective processes that will later become 'psychology' (Goldstein 2003: 131).

A natural history of seeing: Buffon and tactile vision

Even in an age of grand projects like Diderot and d'Alembert's 28-volume *Encyclopédie*, that of their contemporary George-Louis Leclerc, Comte de Buffon was impressive. His *Histoire naturelle, générale et particulière* (known as the *Natural History*), written between 1749 and 1788, was published in thirty-six volumes. His other output in mathematics, bio-geography and natural history was also prodigious. He corresponded with Gabriel Cramer, a Fellow of the Royal Society, and others on topics of mechanics, geometry, probability, number theory, and the differential and integral calculus. His reputation was built through publications such as *Discours sur la manière d'étudier et de traiter l'histoire naturelle*, a work of methodological exposition that worked as the proper introduction to the *Natural History*, known as the *Premier discours*, as well as *Théorie de la terre* and *Histoire des animaux*, all three of which were published in 1749. Buffon's intention was to publish fifty volumes of his *Histoire naturelle* but only thirty-six had appeared by the time of his death. The scope of the project was remarkable, attempting to present all knowledge of natural history, the great length of geological time, and anthropology and their interconnections in a systematic way, being among the first to create an autonomous science free from theological influence. Lyon summarises the impact of the work in no uncertain terms: 'Buffon's *Histoire Naturelle* has been called the *De Rerum Natura* of the eighteenth century' (1976: 133). Indeed, like Lucretius' epic poem which explained the mechanisms through which the cosmos and life unfolded, Buffon also questioned the fixity of the categories of species, observed similarities between related animals, and was acknowledged by Darwin as invoking an early incarnation of evolutionary theory (see e.g. Bowler 2003).

Buffon shared with Diderot not only an interest in the transmutation of species but also a belief in the material origin of life as opposed to supernatural intervention. But whereas Diderot's speculations on the matter occurred in rather poetic and feverishly speculative form in his *Le Rêve de d'Alembert* ['D'Alembert's dream'] (1769), Buffon's style and approach was resolutely scientific. The *Premier discours* demonstrated that he had envisioned the nature of science and scientific method, and also understood the connections between palaeontology, zoological geography, and animal psychology. His appointment as the Intendant at the Jardin du roi in Paris in 1739 led to the gardens significantly increasing in size and transformed them into a major research centre, now a department of the Muséum National d'Histoire Naturelle. Buffon remained there for the rest of his life, being in a position to devote himself to the multi-volume publication.

If his output was prodigious, however, not everyone agreed that his reputation was comparable to Lucretius. Buffon was in fact snubbed by mathematicians, chemists, and astronomers and, despite his great contributions to natural history, his fellow naturalists offered little support, some even reproaching him for an ostentatious and over-complicated writing style. An extra sting perhaps would be felt in criticisms from the brightest stars of the intellectual firmament:

> Though the public was nearly unanimous in its admiration of him, he met with numerous detractors among the learned. The theologians were aroused by his conceptions of geological history; others criticized his views on biological classification; the philosopher Etienne de Condillac disputed his views on the mental faculties of animals; and many took from his work only some general philosophical ideas about nature that were not faithful to what he had written. Voltaire did not appreciate his style, and d'Alembert called him 'the great phrasemonger'. (Piveteau 1995)

Irrespective of issues of style, one potential factor in his negative reception was his resolutely scientific and systematic approach to matters of nature. Against the background of his critics' anthropocentric spirit of Enlightenment inquiry, the *Histoire naturelle* places consideration of the human species in volume IV. It is in chapter 6 of that volume in particular, 'On the sense of seeing', that Buffon directly engages with his contemporaries in terms of philosophical and physiological approaches to vision and its relationship with touch. To the reader acquainted with Voltaire's *Éléments*, published ten years earlier, much material would seem familiar. Not only is there discussion of Cheselden's cataract surgery (his name is spelled 'Chesselden' in J. S. Barr's 1797 English translation) and the observations of restored sight, but one of Voltaire's examples of visual illusion is also alluded to here, the instance of seeing cylindrical towers clearly, but not distinctly, from afar.

What links Voltaire and Buffon is not simply a thematic overlap, nor coverage of similar examples of blindness and vision. Instead, they share a more scientifically developed approach. Whereas Voltaire was interested in exploring optics and the mechanics of vision in a book predominantly concerned with a popularisation of Newtonian physics, Buffon unsurprisingly takes a more biological approach, placing the mechanics of human vision only in terms of longer-term patterns in natural history, among extended discussion of such subjects as puberty, old age, and the characteristics of different races of peoples around the world. Buffon's intention in the chapter 'On the sense of seeing' was not just to familiarise a scientifically inclined general readership with cataract surgery and the trope of the blind man with restored vision. Rather, his wider contribution lay in interpreting the material in terms of neonatal development. Buffon's eye for natural history is productively lent to this previously familiar material such that, early in the chapter, he remarks on the perceptual abilities of the newly born infant and observes how the more complex organs involved in perception, with the greater number of nerve endings, develop sooner *in utero*: 'the parts of the body which are furnished with the greatest quantity of nerves, as the ears and eyes, are those which first appear, and which are soonest brought to perfection' (Buffon 1797: 138). By refracting previous discussions on vision through the lens of neonatal development, Buffon does more than place human mechanisms and the development of vision within an extended natural history context. In other hands, where writing truths allows strategic fictions, one approach would be to invoke another artful invention, an alternative hypothetical blank-blind figure who must learn how to see: neither Diderot's *aveugle-né* (the man born blind), nor his pre-social *muet de convention*, nor even Condillac's statue coming to life, but a hypothetical neonate, a newborn who must make sense of seeing. But Buffon is too scientific, too methodologically aware, more keen on surveying and cataloguing natural phenomena than on teasing out truths from playful philosophical speculation. Nevertheless, how Buffon conceptualises vision in its relation to, and continual interaction with, touch from birth onwards is instructive for the literature on blindness. As readers, we might adopt the strategy of fancifully superimposing such a hypothetical blank-blind neonate figure on to Buffon's chapter on seeing right from the start, for it unfolds in almost chronological developmental fashion, starting with newborns, increasing the correlations between vision and touch through the coordination of the hands, the learning of perspective and then a stronger thesis arguing for sight as a form of touch, and finally dealing with the resolution of visual illusions.

Shortly after birth, the hypothetical neonate shows no 'consistency' of vision, the eyes do not fix on objects, and 'rays of light strike but confusedly on the retina' (Buffon 1797: 139). Descartes had earlier proved through experimentation with a bull's eyeball, first, that the lens fixes the angles of light through the eye and, secondly, that the image that arrives on to the back of the retina is inverted. Thus the retinal image is both double and inverted, as Buffon reminds us, but this is remedied through 'the practice of handling different objects' and 'custom induces them to believe they see objects in the position the touch represents them to the mind' (1797: 139). From this early stage in the chapter, and also in the life of the neonate, the necessity for the repeated correlation of vision and touch, retinal image and haptic sensation, is established. Likewise, if an object is placed close enough to our nose, this double nature of the image becomes apparent and its position indeterminate, so that it is by touching the object, again, that we definitively know of its position in space. In this case, if the retinal image is doubled and then resolved into one, we can understand that 'our imagination forms them single' (1797: 141). When this happens, even as adults, we obtain a glimpse once again of how vision in earlier developmental stages works, accommodating other sensory input in order to learn how to see once again. To shore up this analogy Buffon turns to another case of the surgeon 'Chesselden'. The surgeon had explained how a man had suffered a blow to the head which resulted in squinting and double vision. Through renewed correlation with other senses, these double images slowly but deliberately became resolved once again into a single object. Does this not incontrovertibly demonstrate, says Buffon, that 'in reality [i.e. the retinal image] we see things double, and that it is by habit alone we conceive them to be single' (1797: 142)?

Cheselden's report of couching cataracts and restoring vision is recounted by Buffon, but he leads up to it by speculating how, through the eyes of a hypothetical neonate, we commonly order visual sensations according to perspective, and come to recognise objects outside the body. Buffon proposes that this becomes habitual through the correlations of hand and eye, and consequently that the hand is, in his words, 'constantly measuring':

> By the sense of seeing we can form no idea of distances; without aided by the touch [sic], every object would appear to be within our eyes; and an infant, that is as yet a stranger to the sense of feeling

[i.e. not yet correlating sight with touch], must conceive that every thing it sees exists within itself. The objects only appear to be more or less bulky as they approach to or recede from the eye; insomuch that a fly near the eye will appear larger than an ox at a distance. It is experience alone that can rectify this mistake; and it is by constantly measuring with the hand, and removing from one place to another, that children obtain ideas of distance and magnitude. (1797: 143)

Like Condillac's statue in the *Traité*, which when it opens its eyes initially has no sense of space, distance, or the relative size of an external object, and must depend on touch to open out its world, Buffon's neonate resolves the flat, inverted, and double retinal images into solid and scaled objects by reaching out and touching them. The rather superficial observation by Cheselden of his patient, repeated elsewhere, that on opening his eyes for the first time objects seemed to touch his eyes is at least partially placed into context. On the one hand, Cheselden had written: 'When he first saw, he was so far from making any Judgment about Distances, that he thought all Objects whatever touch'd his Eyes (as he express'd it)' (1728: 448). On the other hand, Buffon's recounting of Cheselden's report restates what facts are present while embellishing certain aspects:

At first the operation was performed only upon one of his eyes, and when he saw for the first time, so far was he from judging distances, that he supposed (as he himself expressed it) every thing he saw touched his eyes, in the same manner as every thing he felt touched his skin. (1797: 145)

In light of Condillac's statue or a hypothetical neonate, the distinction is made between the flat space of the retinal image, where patterns of light form and float seemingly before the eyes, and the process of resolving these into external objects, separate from one's own body, that the body perceives and interacts with. Buffon reminds us that the process took Cheselden's patient two months, and highlights the crucial role of the hand, and of active touching, in the formation of the concomitant concepts of perspective, distance, shape, and size. Even if Buffon is primarily re-articulating Berkeley's position, and though Voltaire had articulated a similar concern with 'Figure', 'Magnitude', and 'Distance', the reader appraises the argument through, as it were, the eyes, and indeed hands, of the neonate. In revisiting Cheselden's report, Buffon reveals to his readers the factors most of interest to his natural history approach, and perhaps given the *Premier discours*' focus on scientific methodology, he starts by framing this familiar material through a more rigidly scientific perspective. We might remember that the full title of Cheselden's report to the Royal Society included the words 'who was born blind, or who lost his sight so early, that he had no remembrance of ever having seen, and was couch'd between 13 and 14 years of age'. Buffon dispels any assumption by the reader that Cheselden's patient was strictly blind in both eyes, and explains that the patient was able to distinguish light from dark and therefore had basic light perception, although no ability to discern an object's shape; he also reminds his readers that the operations on each eye were separated by a year. From Buffon's adopted scientific perspective, in other words, this was not the revelatory moment of seeing the world for the first time that his more romantically inclined countrymen had rhapsodised about and dramatically heightenened.

Nevertheless, elsewhere within Buffon's recounting there remains an unusual mixture of scientific detachment and earnest wonder. The experience of Cheselden's patient seeing a painting on a wall, and examining a miniature portrait within a watch-case, has been discussed previously in relation to Cheselden and the idea of touching with the eyes. However, some measure of Buffon's fascination about the ideas of sight and scale come across in his account, as 'we cannot judge the magnitude of objects but by the largeness of the angle, or rather the image, which they form in our eyes' (1797: 148) and so we are easily deceived in terms of scale. For example, when the patient was shown his mother's pocket watch with a portrait inlaid of his father, in Buffon's words 'he readily perceived the resemblance, yet he expressed his amazement how so large a face could be comprised in so small a compass; to him it seemed as strange as that a pint vessel should contain a bushel' (1797: 146). This confusion of scale persisted such that he also failed to comprehend how the small apartment he dwelt in could be situated inside a larger house. But other, unscientific curiosities emerge in Buffon's reporting, as when a walk in the dark woods by a sighted man offers up shapes that the eye must interpret. A glimpse of a broken tree branch may yield imaginations of more fantastical objects, and again scale is indeterminate – at least, until 'he approaches it and knows it by feeling', when the 'tremendous form' that it seemed to the walker is now resolved into its 'real and absolute form' (1797: 150), underlining the necessity for touch to instruct vision in terms of scale. The eye allows us to assess the form of the object, but magnitude is relative to other factors. Cheselden's patient has an advantage therefore, as his blindness 'allows him to walk in the night with more confidence and security' (1797: 147). On the one hand, what cannot be seen certainly cannot be suggestive of other forces. On the other, there is a renewed sense of pleasure in his new-found powers of sight. 'No sooner, however, had he begun to enjoy this new sense than he was transported beyond measure; he declared every new object was a new source of delight, and that his pleasure was so great he had not language to express it' (1797: 147).

From early examinations of two-dimensional paintings to the broad and sweeping downs of Epsom, where Cheselden's patient lived and recuperated next, his visual capacities and appreciations continued apace, and some of the patient's enthusiasm seems to be exhibited by Buffon. Somewhat curiously, though, we return to where we began in this book. For Buffon is mindful throughout of the significance of touch in the formation of visual perceptions, to the extent that the crowning insight towards the end of this essay on blindness and seeing inevitably involves tactility. Being acquainted with Descartes' naive conceptualisation of blind men seeing with their hands, the natural historian Buffon now articulates a similar analogy, one which Diderot would explicitly reference in his *Lettre sur les aveugles* soon afterwards, namely, an equivalence between sight and touch that is most evident in cases of blindness:

> We may fairly consider sight as a species of touching, though very different from what we commonly understand by that sense; for in order to excite the latter we must be near the object, whereas we can touch with the eye as far as the light the object contains will make an impression, or its figure form an angle therein. (1797: 152)

However, although we might consider Buffon as returning to Descartes' comfortable analogy, our conceptual starting point, there is additionally an acknowledgement of a form of perception that lies prior to these separate yet related modalities, a model of perception that involves contact in some form, a base tactility, even something that resembles or invokes those Middle Eastern formulations of vision as a form of intromission, such as that of Al-Kindi. Buffon's restless and systematic scientific inquiry has offered up ideas of blindness that are at once dated and familiar, but also wondrous and instructive, and he points to another realm of inquiry and methodological approach in order to pursue this further. We now jog ahead of ourselves chronologically. But thematically, we have set up a framework for contextualising the monumental text in this area of blindness, sensation and language. It is to Diderot's *Lettre sur les aveugles*, and the possibility of a uniquely tactile language, that we now turn.

Chapter 5

The Testimony of Blind Men: Diderot's *Lettre*

> When a blind man speaks, things suddenly become clear. (De Fontenay 1982: 169)

If Voltaire had provided an 'extensive exposition' of the Molyneux problem, offering thin medical reports to uphold a confirmation of Berkeley's philosophical position, less than a decade later Denis Diderot made it, in Cassirer's words, the 'central point of his first psychological and epistemological essay' (1979: 109), the famous *Lettre sur les aveugles, á l'usage de ceux qui voient* ['Letter on the blind, for the benefit of those who see'] (1749). The second clause of the title adds an important qualification to the already established Enlightenment fascination with blindness and 'the man born blind restored to light', as Foucault (2003: 78) expressed it. Unlike Voltaire's invocation of medical reports to justify prior epistemological speculation, Diderot looks to first-person testimony to answer Molyneux's question, but also to develop inherited philosophical wisdom on the subject of blindness.

Diderot's *Lettre* is regarded as his first mature work of philosophy. Descartes and Locke had discounted the complex phenomenology of blindness in order to use the hypothetical blind man as a placeholder for epistemological arguments. Conversely, Diderot was interested in actual experiences of blindness, aiming to interrogate how blind men conceived or grasped the world and reasoned through objects. His *Lettre* was the first of two influential epistolary investigations into sensory impairment that, along with Condillac, helped to advance sensationism in France and differentiate it somewhat from its empiricist influences, particularly Locke and Berkeley. Consequently, the *Lettre* only engages with the Molyneux question towards the end and adds little to that particular debate, and Diderot resists the temptation to investigate further reports of cataract operations on the blind since Grant and Cheselden. Instead, he did something no previous philosopher had done. He departed the Parisian salons and coffeehouses he frequented and actively sought blind men to interrogate. The recorded testimony of blind subjects on the Molyneux question was patchy, so Diderot stressed that his subjects were real, not hypothetical, blind men (in Morgan 1977: 32; Kennedy et al. 1992: 176), and thereby took a step towards redressing the tradition that considered the blind subject as merely a passive object of scrutiny. 'As such,' suggests Curran, 'Diderot liberates the discussion from the confines of an experiment seeking to bring the unseeing into phase with *les voyants* [the sighted]. Instead, he brings *those who see* into phase with the blind' (2000: 77, original emphasis).

Even Diderot's subtitle suggests a straightforward reversal of previous philosophical treatments, such that now 'the blind were to guide the seeing' and, something borne out throughout the *Lettre*, by focusing on actual experience the sighted philosopher may 'enable the seeing philosopher to understand the Other, the blind person, in the latter's own terms' (Paulson 1987: 71). Or such, at least, was the intention. For Diderot to take this stance he had to acknowledge, unlike his British empiricist influences, that 'blindness does not offer a direct solution to the problems of vision, and the seeing do not provide a model with which to imagine and understand the blind' (Paulson 1987: 70). Who could have foreseen that the result of these interviews would be not only the anonymous publication of the *Lettre*, but also a scandal in France and eventually a prison sentence for its author? Diderot's *Lettre* is a non-linear, at times rambling, but mostly perceptive essay that seeks to answer speculative epistemologies about touch and vision through tangible evidence, supposedly collected from actual blind subjects. This is why it 'is referred to by authorities as the first scientific study of the blind' (Davis 1960: 401). Those 'authorities' included the blind professor Pierre Villey, author of *The World of the Blind: A Psychological Study* (1930), and Gabriel Farrell, a director at the Perkins Institute for the Blind, the New England based institution that taught Helen Keller. The *Lettre* would come to be regarded not only as one of the earliest sustained works of philosophical significance on blindness, but also as the beginnings of a more scientific psychological inquiry into blind experience. However, this was not for the reasons that we might think.

One of the most substantial arguments in the *Lettre* concerns signs, and it calls for the development of a distinct and systematic language for the blind, a 'clear and precise language of touch'

(Diderot 1916a: 90).¹ The various writing systems for the blind in existence before the universal adoption of Braille a century later were imprecise. A more systematic language based around touch within the communication process would, Diderot argued, also be useful in communicating with the deaf and deaf-mute. As we shall see, the questions opened up initially by Molyneux about translation between sense modalities, and pursued by Voltaire and Diderot with regard to the specificity of tactile signs and haptic experience for the blind, would become formative for the development of twentieth- and twenty-first-century technological mediations of touch such as Braille readers, tactile-visual substitution systems (TVSS), and the BrainPort™ of Paul Bach-y-Rita. Back in the eighteenth century, after Voltaire's take on blindness based on the Molyneux question and Cheselden's patient, Diderot pursues an unusual and non-linear trajectory concerning blindness, touch, and tactile signs.

The context and the controversy

At one stage in the *Lettre* Diderot writes of his experience of visiting and interviewing an actual blind man in the small French town of Puiseaux, south of Paris. Asked whether he would be overjoyed if he ever regained the use of his eyes, Diderot reports the unnamed blind man as replying:

> I would just as soon have long arms: it seems to me that my hands would tell me more about what happens on the moon than you can find out with your eyes and your telescopes; and besides, eyes cease to see sooner than hands to touch. I would be as well off if I perfected the organ I possess, as if I obtained the organ which I am deprived of. (Diderot 1916a: 77)

Diderot advances prior epistemological debates about blindness, vision, and touch by supposedly looking to empirical sources of evidence, in this case the report of a blind man himself, and there is a genuine fascination with how the blind conceive of vision and visual concepts including distance. Upon further familiarisation with the

---

¹ Throughout this book the standard 1916 translation by Margaret Jourdain has been used. Kate Tunstall's 2011 translation, published by Continuum, which includes a comprehensive essay on blindness and Enlightenment, would now be the preferred translation. However, work on this chapter had started prior to the publication of her book. Her essay is cited several times in this chapter.

Lettre, however, we start to question the validity of such testimony, the point of intersection of authorial text and interviewee's voice.

In the above passage the blind man seems quickly to discount any Cartesian equivalence of hands and eyes, and re-voices Berkeley's position on the incommensurability of visual and tactile space. Knowing that the moon was far away, and consequently that the eye could gain no direct knowledge of it, this man asserts the value of touch as a more reliable path to knowledge. Taken out of context, the passage would seem a succinct and apposite empirical counterpoint to prior epistemological musings on blindness and the space of touch. As readers we might consider this somewhat contrived, crafted around prior philosophical categories of the relationship between vision and touch, an imaginary of blindness by the sighted perhaps. For, in other passages about other blind men, it is not they but Diderot who is revealed, not only in terms of his own philosophical and, it turns out, religious views on the subject of blindness, but also in terms of a positively mercurial narrative and as a dangerously disingenuous voice. Over the course of the letter, conflicting impulses towards blindness are revealed. As Curran explains, 'For the majority of the text, the blind are normalized – explained, rationalized, brought into phase with the reader's notion of normalcy', but elsewhere, conversely, 'the blind are also identified as conceptually other, as anomalous, even monstrous' (2000: 75).

How Diderot came to write an essay that supposedly marks the start of the author's mature and original philosophy, while also signifying a break from deism, and subsequently ended up in prison after its publication is an eye-opening tale in itself. The essay was published anonymously in June 1749, and the authorities tried to suppress its circulation. According to Jonathan Israel's *Radical Enlightenment* (2002), Diderot had already been under police surveillance since 1747 and was soon identified as the author. He then 'had his manuscripts confiscated, and was imprisoned for some months [...] at Vincennes, where he was visited almost daily by Rousseau, at the time his closest and most assiduous ally' (Israel 2002: 710). His eventual release was due to the intervention of Madame du Châtelet, a well-known intellectual figure who translated and interpreted Newton's *Principia mathematica* (and was incidentally one of Voltaire's mistresses), who swayed the prison governor (Morley 1878: 75). How did this come about – the author as mischievous, intriguing, and ultimately scandalous while simultaneously providing one of the most sustained philosophical treatments of blindness in history?

Diderot starts the *Lettre* probably with an awareness that La Mettrie's unambiguously Godless and infamous materialist treatise *L'Homme machine* ['The man machine'] (1748) had been condemned and burned. This might explain the more private and conversational letter form that Diderot adopted; the work is addressed at the beginning to an unnamed 'Madame', and at the end it is signed enigmatically '***', rather than 'Diderot' or 'M. Diderot', as the reader might expect. Tunstall has suggested that 'Madame' may be a fictional convention, or if a real person, either Diderot's mistress, Madame de Puisieux, or perhaps the mathematician Madame de Prémontval, to whom he had dedicated an earlier work (Tunstall 2011: 16). Tunstall makes much of the continual interplay between fact and fiction in the *Lettre*, and the letter form, along with the significant portions of reported speech attributed to the blind subjects, would help ensure that any potentially seditious views expressed were distanced from the author. Yet the *Lettre* turned out to be 'the last [work] in which Diderot the moralist and philosopher tried to express his opinions with any degree of freedom' according to Cru (1913: 154), and further distancing mechanisms are certainly present in the almost hallucinatory materialist meditation *La Rêve d'Alembert* ('D'Alembert's dream', written 1769 but published posthumously).

If the *Lettre* initially reads like an essay in psychology, its meandering nature takes it elsewhere, and Arthur Wilson considers it more as a piece of creative improvisation than a structured essay. It is 'a disarming book, written with the seeming artlessness of someone idly improvising on a musical instrument. One subject suggests another, so that the reader, led on and on through a steeplechase over most of the various metaphysical jumps, finally gets himself soaked in the waterhole called "Does God Exist"?' (Wilson 1972: 97). If Wilson prefers the more rigid and formal compositions of a figure such as J. S. Bach, perhaps, what Diderot offers is more innovative and astonishingly wide-ranging, a disjointed Romantic composition that evinces various moods and shifting tones. Diderot acknowledges this himself at one point. 'We have wandered far from the blind, you will say. True, madam, but you must be so good as to allow me these digressions; I promised you a conversation, and I cannot keep my word without this indulgence' (1916a: 105). Like *La Rêve d'Alembert*, then, the *Lettre* involves a playful and potentially atheistic materialist manifesto, a materialism that imaginatively pushes for an explanation of how matter becomes organised into self-sustaining living beings, and it could be considered a kind of proto-evolutionary theory. The lively dance of ideas around a series of core blind figures is briskly paced and compelling, but sometimes at the expense of a sustained study of blindness in its actuality. Whether dealing with the supposedly real but unnamed blind man of Puiseaux, or the blind mathematician Nicholas Saunderson, who it turns out had died a decade prior to publication, there is a mixture of high-minded metaphysical speculation, digression, and sometimes condescending small-scale observations about sensation without sight, all finding expression through the supposed testimony of a series of blind men.

The free-ranging nature of the *Lettre*, and its potentially seditious content, is one reason why Israel considers it a unique and significant text, and his summary clearly demonstrates its staunchly anti-Cartesian and radically subversive nature:

> This powerful essay [...] revolves around a remarkable deathbed scene in which a dying blind philosopher, Saunderson, rejects the arguments of a providential God during his last hours. Saunderson's arguments are those of a Neo-Spinozist, Naturalist, and Fatalist, using a sophisticated notion of the self-generation and natural evolution of species without Creation or supernatural intervention. The notion of 'thinking matter' is upheld and the 'argument from design' discarded [...] as hollow and unconvincing. (2002: 710)

As Paulson and others suggest to varying degrees, there are deeply entrenched literary and historical tropes of blindness, explored elsewhere in this book in further detail, which readers of Diderot's *Lettre* might call to mind – associations between blindness as darkness, as death, or as a 'groping approach to truth' (Paulson 1987: 69) which exchanges physiological blindness for some form of inner truth or insight. In other words, Diderot's blind man, especially in the second section on Saunderson, can be at one remove from the sighted reader, a convenient avatar or blank receptacle who is at once a repository for pity and, if not a hypothetical blind man in this instance, a figure who we permit to baldly articulate the author's more controversial religious and metaphysical arguments. As Curran summarises, 'In the *Lettre*, the blind hold a dark mirror in front of us, a mirror in which we perceive the precariousness of our beliefs in physical, esthetic and metaphysical realms' (2000: 78). Against the assumption of certainty, the search for the scientific and philosophical truths of blindness of Hilmer, Cheselden, and Voltaire, Diderot shows the sighted reader how our sense-based conventions of understanding start to unravel when vision is removed from the equation. Diderot will controversially demonstrate that, while the sighted share tactile and olfactory phenomena with the blind, the achievement of a collective humanity, a shared sense of endeavour, a sense of unity within the cosmos, and a divine order assumes the power of sight. With a mixture of caution and eagerness, we should bear this in mind as we embark upon a closer reading of Diderot's *Lettre*.

For the benefit of those who see: the argument of the *Lettre*

The *Lettre* begins by being rather dismissive about the fascination with the surgical restoration of sight so in vogue at the time, instead offering an earnest investigation into the psychology of the blind, questioning actual blind subjects about their experience. Rather than commencing with Diderot's perspective on the Molyneux question, the first section of the *Lettre* involves an interview with the unnamed blind man in the town of Puiseaux, questioned on the effect of the absence of one sense on the formation of metaphysical and moral ideas. The second section then documents another blind subject's fatalistic musings on the existence of God and the possibility of a self-creating and self-sustaining universe, in so doing voicing the author's own metaphysical concerns. Finally, the essay turns to the more familiar and sober discussion of the Molyneux problem, Cheselden's patient, and the origin and formation of ideas through the senses, becoming a more conventional text in terms of its contribution to sensationism.

Diderot starts from the knowingly naive but firm position that 'the state of our organs and our senses has a great deal of influence on our metaphysics and ethics', and that 'that great proof (of God's existence) derived from the wonders of nature is very weak for blind people' (1916a: 80). Along the lines of a naive sensationist epistemology, and extending the licence of the British empiricists' concentration on experience, Diderot's initial assumption is that complex metaphysical arguments are more difficult for the blind as, like the man of Puiseaux who wishes to touch the moon with his long arms, the building blocks of sensation are of a different type. A sensory impairment such as blindness or deafness affords an opportunity for a sensationist in their inquiry to consider an alternative, non-normative sensorium, and this is irresistible for Diderot. 'We only distinguish the presence of external things from their picture in our imagination by the strength or weakness of the impression; and similarly, the blind only distinguish the sensation from the actual presence of an object at their fingers' ends, by the strength or weakness of that sensation' (1916a: 86). Whether or not the blind subjects voiced such arguments, and to what extent they served as characters within a semi-fictional thought experiment, is open to question. But in a follow-up text in the same spirit, *Lettre sur les sourds et muets* ['Letter on the deaf and dumb'] (1751), Diderot was equally keen to pursue the mechanisms behind the formation of metaphysical ideas through divergent sensory epistemologies. As an 1899 essay on the Encyclopaedists summarises, 'Diderot attempted, as Condillac did afterwards, to work out the psychological development of sensationalism' (Lévy-Bruhl 1899: 139). Questioning how a blind person might conceive of proofs of the existence of God based upon final causes is one way to pursue this. 'Cheselden's experiment and Molyneux's problem were known,' Lévy-Bruhl continues; 'Diderot wished to go beyond these, to carry this kind of "metaphysical anatomy" still farther, and to take in pieces, so to speak, the senses of man' (1899: 139).

At times Diderot falls back into the well-worn and now over-familiar trope of marvelling at the non-visual capacities and coping mechanisms of the blind, remarking on the heightened tactile sensitivity by which Saunderson could tell coins apart by means of the fingertips, the Puiseaux man's conception of the moon's distance from us, or how a blind man envisions or imagines a mirror in tactile terms. Such low-level observations fail to advance the philosophical arguments, and seem to pander to the curiosity and prejudices of the sighted readership. Upon Diderot asking his interlocutor what a mirror is, for example, the blind man replies: 'An instrument [...] which sets things in relief at a distance from themselves, when properly placed in regard to it. It is like my hand, which, to feel an object, I must not put on one side of it' (1916a: 71). In fact Diderot is pleased with this answer, saying: 'Had Descartes been born blind, he might, I think, have hugged himself for such a definition' (1916a: 72). Perhaps so. But these low-level insights into the blind man's world of perception lure the inquisitive, sighted reader into larger, more dangerous speculative territories altogether, the kinds of 'intellectual excesses' that Pierre-Nicholas Berryer noted in a letter to the Count d'Argenson, the man who eventually ordered Diderot to jail in Vincennes according to Wilson (1972: 103–4). Notwithstanding the darkness and inconvenience of prison, the curious sighted were not the only beneficiaries of the *Lettre*, as the scandal indirectly drew attention to the plight of the blind in France. 'If, as Marie-Jean Hérault de Séchelles wrote, Diderot's conversation was like a beautiful flame that drew any number of objects,' summarises Weygand, 'they were certainly well and truly illuminated' (2009: 68).

Notwithstanding the idiosyncratic style which Wilson compared unfavourably to music, the flickering beautiful flame did indeed shed light on the significance of touch to the blind in more abstract ways. Diderot's interview with the second blind man, the mathematician Nicholas Saunderson, revealed his system of palpable arithmetic and thereby how touch alone could 'produce a system of abstract signs identical to that produced by the clear-sighted' (Weygand 2009: 68). It was this discussion around the centrality of touch in the *Lettre* that led to the recognition of the fundamental role of touch, and the assertion of its pre-eminence over sight, in the *Natural History* of Buffon, who lauded 'the fine and lively metaphysics' of Diderot's *Lettre*, and in Condillac's *Traité des sensations*.

The blind man of Puiseaux

The *Lettre* commences with some apologetic scene-setting, for Diderot had petitioned for an invitation from a Monsieur René-Antoine de Réaumur to his parlour, where he hoped to be present at a demonstration of restored sight in the manner made famous by Cheselden in 1728. A Prussian surgeon named Hilman had been invited to perform the couching operation on a girl born blind, the daughter of a man named Simoneau. The unbandaging ceremony would be a significant event, an entertainment for a curious intellect. Unfortunately, despite repeated requests, Réaumur chose not to invite Diderot and so it would be other, less qualified eyes (rather dismissively 'quelques yeux sans consequence' in the original, denoting mediocre minds) that would be present after the operation, not those of a trained and appreciative *philosophe* like Diderot. The self-conscious theatricality of the unbandaging event, a staged spectacle for those sighted attendees, is frustratingly denied to Diderot. As Paulson explains, 'the moment of first sight, which Foucault calls the rediscovery of the childhood gaze, is also a magical apparition or raising of a curtain' (1987: 41). Foucault had identified 'the man born blind restored to light' as the foundational myth of the Enlightenment, with its promise of a rediscovery of 'the permanent birth of truth' through the 'bright, distant, open naivety of the gaze' (Foucault 2003: 78). The dramatic component of the great reveal would be compelling to anyone, but especially so for a *philosophe* with an interest in the origins of human knowledge through sensation. So, on the day of the operation, swallowing his pride, Diderot left Paris for the small town of Puiseaux to interview an *aveugle-né*, a man born blind. This blind subject remains anonymous throughout, Diderot travelling to the provinces, in his words, to 'have some talk with the Puiseaux man who was born blind' (1916a: 69). If Diderot is denied the satisfaction of his philosophical curiosity through visual spectacle, he will attain it through other means.

As we have seen, hypothetical speculations on the epistemology of blindness abounded, especially in the absence of rigorous scientific findings. Non-standardised approaches to recording data from surgery, coupled with the difficulty of categorising the level of visual impairment of the patients, or even whether they were congenitally or adventitiously blind, were compounded by other factors. In France, Voltaire's recounting of Cheselden's ocular surgery in 1728 had clearly drawn the attention of other sensationist philosophers, in a manner consistent with Foucault's identification of the moment of first sight. Despite the Molyneux question having been pitted in 1688, the mythical aspect remained, while the accumulating evidence was messy or inconclusive. La Mettrie, in his *Treatise of the Soul* (1745), and then Condillac in his *Essay on the Origin of Human Knowledge* (1746), were wise to this, critiquing available data and judging the partiality of Cheselden's experiment. 'By dint of tormenting the newly sighted man,' wrote La Mettrie for example, 'they got him to say what they wanted to hear' (in Weygand 2009: 60). The naivety involved in the trope of the blind gaze being newly restored to sight remained unchallenged. But Diderot's *Lettre* surely had a role in demystifying blindness through the testimony of the blind men, the son of a philosopher in Puiseaux and the mathematics professor Saunderson, so that the 'common' blind could be shown as neither intellectually nor spiritually inferior. This aspect of public understanding of blindness would be crucial in the story of the first schools for the blind, detailed in the following chapter.

A shift in the sighted public's imaginary of the sighted was starting to take place. Hitherto, the blind were presumed incapable of deceiving, were literally in contact with truth through touching, yet could easily be misled or tricked by the unscrupulous sighted. This public perception of the blind as childlike innocents would slowly be reconsidered as a result of the growing awareness, through written accounts and theatrical demonstrations, of ocular surgery, and the blind men's testimony in the *Lettre* could only benefit this slow process of demystification. As Weygand puts it, 'the progress of ocular surgery, despite the failures due to lack of asepsis, antisepsis, and anaesthesia, contributed to the desacralization of blindness, which began to be viewed as a curable ailment and not as a sign of insurmountable difference' (2009: 62). Although sometimes still marked as benignly different through their proven strength of memory and capacity for abstract thought, the rights of the blind to share in the benefits of literacy would gather strength, and a wave of interest arose in late eighteenth-century Paris to enable them to share in the fruits of the Enlightenment. But until 1749, if no-one had actually met or become acquainted with a blind person, stories circulating about blindness were often apocryphal or curiously non-specific.

Into this situation Diderot introduces the nameless 'blind man of Puiseaux'. The initial questions put to him are not exactly scientific, encompassing a salacious fascination with what this blind man may find beautiful, questioning the possibility of morality in the blind, and introjecting a propensity for abstraction including increased mathematical and geometrical abilities and even timekeeping. Given his inability to be present at the cataract operation and its immediate revelatory aftermath, Diderot consoles himself by justifying the philosophical redundancy of the drama, instead stressing the utility of understanding how the blind ordinarily perceive. Whether this further essentialises 'blindness' as an entirely separate mode of perceiving and experiencing the world from the sighted, or helps to 'normalise' blind experience so the sighted get to apprehend the world otherwise, remains an unresolved tension. However, Diderot's questioning process does develop into a self-proclaimed scientific, indeed psychological, endeavour:

> People try to give those born blind the gift of sight, but rightly considered, science would be equally advanced by questioning a sensible blind man. We should learn to understand his psychology and should compare it with ours, and perhaps we should thereby come to a solution of the difficulties that make the theory of vision and of the senses so intricate and confused [...] To train and question one born blind would be an occupation worthy of the combined talents of Newton, Descartes, Locke and Leibniz. (Diderot 1916a: 116–18)

This is a noble enterprise when articulated in this way, as it is towards the end of the *Lettre*. But Diderot's questioning of the apparently sensible blind man from Puiseaux in the first part initially fails to live up to this standard. The casually curious sighted reader is lured into the text through reassuring means, Diderot being quick to offer the kinds of comparisons between the blind and the sighted that might confirm the commonsense suspicions of the sighted. For this blind man, at least according to Diderot, beauty is judged through touch, hearing is more acute, the experience of time passing is more accurately measured and, intriguingly, his arms and hands work like scales and compasses, being more precise in their judgement of the weight and distance of objects than those of the sighted. Diderot reports that the blind man's father was Professor of Philosophy at the University of Paris, a fact that no doubt conveniently helped establish the credibility of his blind witness as an educated man. He lived the life of a cultured gentleman in the provinces, fully able to articulate how he comprehends the world and acquires knowledge in it, often through forms of sensory translation. Pressed a little by Diderot on exactly how he conceives of visual concepts such as what a mirror is, what an eye does, or what symmetry consists in, the blind man articulates his answers through the familiar mechanism of a sensory analogy. This is why Diderot repeats Descartes' sensory analogy between hands and eyes at this stage in the *Lettre*, for greater authority through the mouth of the blind man from Puiseaux. Try telling the man blind and deaf from birth that 'the head is the seat of our thoughts' (1916a: 87), for example, and the more tactually-inclined and acoustically aware blind respondent would disagree:

> If ever a philosopher, blind and deaf from his birth, were to construct a man after the fashion of Descartes, I can assure you, madam, that he would put the seat of the soul at the fingers' ends, for thence the greater part of the sensations and all his knowledge are derived. (1916a: 87)

The correspondence between the greater sensitivity of the fingers due to denser nerve endings and the parts of the eye with greater nerve density, the macula and fovea, would be developed later in technologies for the blind that concretised the Puiseaux man's analogy. More abstractly, a blind and deaf subject would utilise touch sensations as the basis or building block for all their more complex ideas – a living prototype for a Lockean empiricist epistemology, in other words. How would the world seem if it were built predominantly through successive tactile sensations? A few years later, this exact question would form the basis for much of Condillac's *Traité des sensations*. For now, Diderot is interested in how this might affect other areas of thought and judgement for the subject, including morality and metaphysics. In her book on Diderot, De Fontenay suggests that he was exploring alternative scenarios to the usual metaphysical privileging of sight, enshrined in Western philosophy since Aristotle's hymn to vision in the first part of his *Metaphysics*. If instead one multiplies the senses and de-hierarchises them, the victor in such a carnival of the senses would be touch:

> It takes over marvellously well for sight and is quick to demonstrate that it needs no help in awakening a man and opening him up to the fullness of the world. This is so much the case that the blind man of Puiseaux hopes for a miracle from neither heaven nor medicine. (De Fontenay 1982: 166)

Even if the blind man were offered the miracle of the restoration of sight, he would reject this outright, familiar as he is with the world of touch. He had explained his reasoning previously: 'eyes cease to see sooner than hands to touch. I would be as well off if I perfected the organ I possess, as if 1 obtained the organ which I am deprived of' (Diderot 1916a: 77).

But another remark from the Puiseaux man suddenly opens up into more philosophical territory, that of the relationship between language and the senses, and the nature of discourse without the benefit of sight. 'I perceive, gentlemen,' says the blind man to Diderot's party at one point, 'that you are not blind: you are astonished at what I do, and why not as much at my speaking?' (1916a: 79). A seemingly innocuous, self-deprecating and even amusing comment slowly opens into a different line of questioning, where the questions and answers centre around language and signs for the blind, and the potential for translatability through the senses. Moving away from any straightforward model of sensory equivalence, Diderot starts to question the translatability of tactile signs into other signs, furthering the argument for abstraction based upon what is intromitted through the sense organs. If marks and symbols are visible to the eye, sounds and utterances audible to the ear, then there is no haptic equivalent for the skin: 'we have none for the sense of touch, even though this sense, too, has its own particular method of speaking and of eliciting responses' (1916a: 89). Diderot's concern here is that perceiving the world through non-visual means is all very well, but if the articulation of that experience involves sensory analogues that misconceive or fail to fully comprehend the function of eyes, mirrors, or symmetry, then other aspects of their intellectual operations may also become suspect. In part this is a function of communication through whatever senses are available, something the sighted take for granted, especially through reading. If there is no communication to one born blind, deaf, and dumb, then they may grow physically, Diderot argues, but will remain in a state of 'imbecility'. This stresses the importance of early communication in 'some fixed, determinate, and consistently uniform way' – that is, a tactile language. Diderot continues: 'in a word, if we were to trace the same letters on their hands that we ourselves draw on paper and if the same meaning were invariably attached to them' (1916a: 89), like any other fixed, determinate sign system, then this would imply a translatability between spatially distributed signs perceived sequentially, and therefore temporally, through the skin as a new form of literacy, a different configuration of sense and sign that is readable by the blind, and facilitated due to their enhanced capacity for abstraction:

> But if the imagination of the blind man be no more than the faculty of calling to mind and combining sensations of palpable points; and of a sighted man, the faculty of combining and calling to mind visible or coloured points, the person born blind consequently perceives things in a much more abstract manner than we [sighted]; and in questions purely speculative, he is perhaps less liable to be deceived. (1916a: 87)

Diderot has already celebrated the ability of the blind to grasp abstractions more ably than the sighted, a commonplace observation. But by considering the role of tactile points in space in the abstraction process, there is added an ability to grasp mathematical and geometric truths with certainty, to further knowledge through the manipulation of signs, letters, and numbers, and therefore to translate effectively between sensory realms. While not exactly a new idea, this remained a powerful and persistent one, demonstrated through the tortuous development of a range of competing tactile writing systems during this period, one of which was documented by Diderot in his 'Addition to the Preceding Letter', which eventually resulted in the adoption of Braille.

The interview with the blind man from Puiseaux is unlikely to be symptomatic of an absolute shift from the blind man as 'object' of philosophical inquiry to his becoming a 'subject' of equal stature, as Weygand claims (2009: 63). But certainly there was some measure of demystification of blindness and blind experience through his testimony. It is difficult to say the same for the next blind man to be interviewed in the *Lettre* who, as many readers would be unaware, had already been dead for ten years by the time it was written. This was no barrier for Diderot's creative prose.

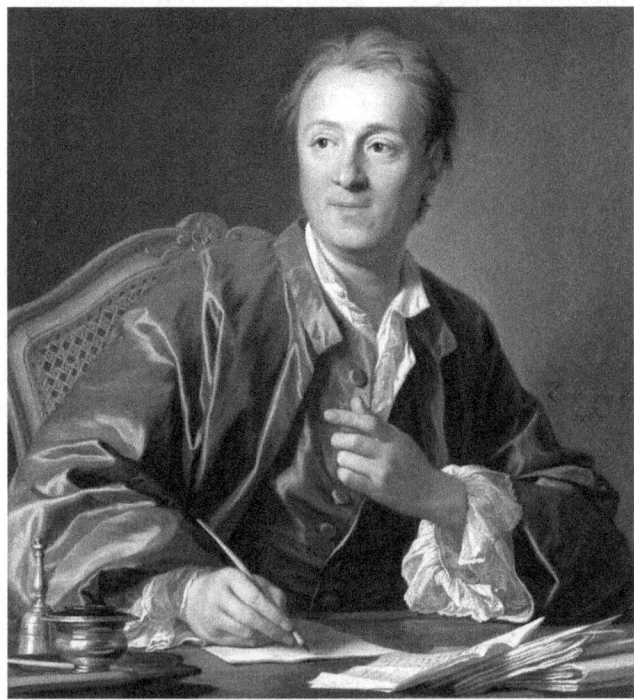

Figure 5.1 Portrait of Denis Diderot by Louis-Michel van Loo, 1767. Louvre Museum, Paris.

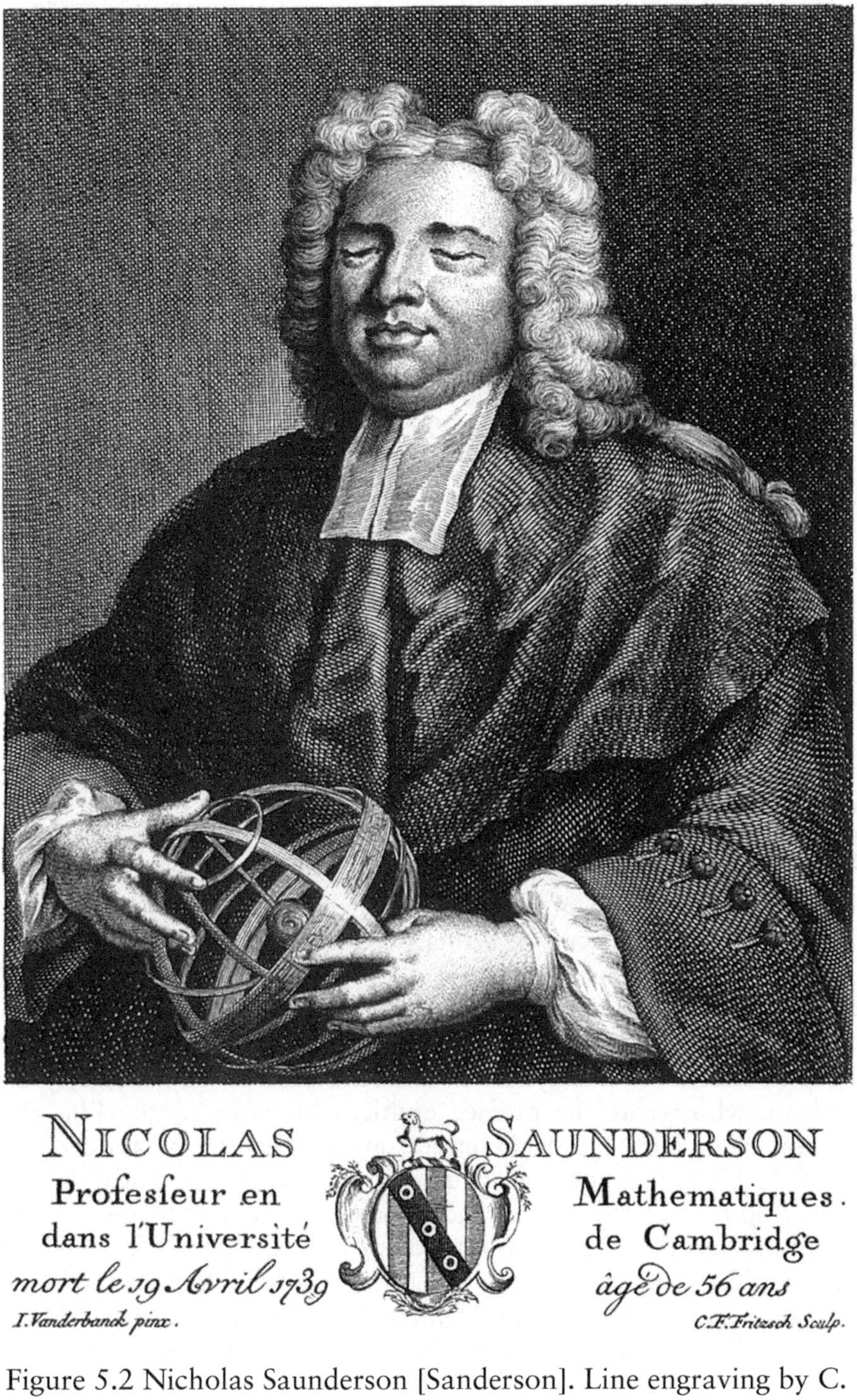

Diderot's Lettre

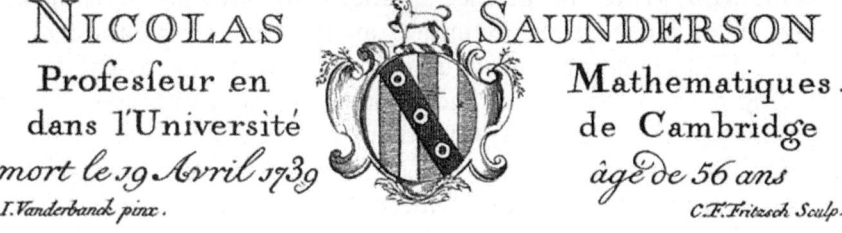

Figure 5.2 Nicholas Saunderson [Sanderson]. Line engraving by C. F. Fritzsch after J. Vanderbank, 1719.

The blind man of numbers

The first blind man had gone beyond any straightforward sensory equivalence between the senses, or analogy between eyes and hands, to assert the prevalence of touch over sight. Furthermore, Diderot had claimed that, true to a sensationist epistemology, the nature of the ideas formed by the blind were different than those of the sighted, and if simple ideas led to more complex ideas, then surely our most complex systems of thought would ultimately be affected. As Diderot put it, 'the state of our organs and our senses has a great deal of influence on our metaphysics and our morality' (1916a: 80). Interested as Diderot was in the blind man's ability to abstract palpable points and signs, and the potential for translation between them, inevitably there would be differences between the worlds of the blind and those of the sighted. In terms of evidencing such differences in morality and religion, Diderot considered that 'perhaps the crucial case might be that of a highly intelligent and gifted blind person' (Davis 1960: 402). The second blind subject in the *Lettre*, the mathematician Nicholas Saunderson, was such a person.

Rather than being yet another unnamed hypothetical blind man, there is a historical record of Saunderson, the Lucasian Professor of Mathematics at Cambridge, blind since the age of twelve months, who had lectured on optics and vision. Lord Chesterfield, who apparently attended some of Saunderson's courses between 1712 and 1714, described him 'as a professor who had not the use of his own eyes, but taught others to use theirs' (in Baker 2007). He was known to be outspoken, and distinguished himself from other Cambridge colleagues and his predecessor, William Whiston, by his lack of interest in theology: 'Whiston was dismissed for having too much religion and Saunderson preferred for having none' (Dyer 1824, in Baker 2007). Saunderson's major book, *The Elements of Algebra*, was published in ten volumes with the help of his successor at Cambridge, John Colson, who wrote the preface entitled 'Memoirs of the Life and Character of Dr. Nicholas Saunderson' the year after Saunderson's death in 1740. Diderot was acquainted with the biographical details, including his theological reticence, and was clearly impressed by the ingenious use that Saunderson made of bespoke marked tablets and rulers in his complex calculations. Here was a living instantiation of the abstract tactile operations Diderot had mentioned earlier in the *Lettre*. 'We only know that his fingers moved over his tablet with astonishing rapidity,' marvelled Diderot of Saunderson, 'that he made the longest calculations successfully; that he could interrupt them, and recognise when he was in error; that he could verify them with ease; and that this work did not take him as much time as one might imagine, because he could arrange his tablet to suit his convenience' (1916a: 96).

The independence that Saunderson demonstrated in terms of perception and cognitive ability greatly excited Diderot, and he perceived a difference both in tactile acuity and cognitive ability between the two blind men. Diderot knew that the earlier conversation with the Puiseaux man, where a mirror was conceived in tactile terms, while amusing to the curious reader, was misconceived. Creech terms this a 'tropological error' in equating the mirror with the hand through tactile means, since of course there is no tactual relief, and so they are quite literally 'palpably different' (1986: 116). By contrast, Diderot says of Saunderson that he 'saw by means of his skin' (1916a: 107), a more developed and independent form of blindness than that of the Puiseaux man, who although he was of independent means, had a more meandering philosophical inclination, and volunteered that he depended on his wife to be his eyes: 'He married to have eyes of his own' (1916a: 79). Conversely, being so adept, Saunderson became one of the inspirations for Enlightenment efforts to raise the intellectual aspirations of the blind. Diderot reasoned that since 'abstraction consists only of separating by thought the sensible qualities of bodies', the blind were at an advantage, so 'the blind man perceives things in a much more abstract manner than we do' (1916a: 82). If, among other things, the *Lettre* reveals Diderot's interest in questions of an empirical protopsychology of the blind, the segment on Saunderson further cements the potential not only for a tactile language, but also for further abstract pursuits such as mathematical operations through haptic manipulation.

Proceeding from the Lockean point that 'our most intellectual ideas [...] are very much dependent on the structure of our body', and consequently that our organs and senses have 'a great deal of influence on our metaphysics and our morality' (1916a: 80), Diderot considered the implications for such philosophical questioning given the removal of sight. If the process of demystification and the investigation of complex ideas starts with the first blind man, the discussion of the second, Saunderson, proceeds even further in that direction, from sensation to abstraction, where numerical calculations and geometry remain consistent despite the absence of vision. Given insufficient, asymmetric, or simply non-visual sensory input, our reasoning is trustworthy in some systematic areas such as mathematics, thinks Diderot, but when applied to other complex areas may lead to flawed metaphysical constructs. Given their altered sensory capabilities, then, Diderot reflects upon how 'that great proof (of God's existence) derived from the wonders of nature is very weak for blind people' (Cru 1913: 155), and so Diderot is at great pains to point out 'the weakness of reasoning from the data of our senses in such a weighty subject' (Cru 1913: 163). After La Mettrie's imprisonment, and mindful of the hostile climate to challenging or dangerous ideas in France at that time, having Saunderson voice controversial theological ideas would surely lead to the conclusion that these were the result of the blind man's flawed reasoning, rather than the views of the author of the *Lettre*.

First of all, in order to demonstrate his witness's credibility, Diderot included a biographical introduction to Saunderson the man and the mathematician. The attentive reader may become aware of substantial slippage between the historical actuality of Saunderson and the character who voices metaphysical doubts and atheistic speculations on his deathbed in Diderot's pages. Having earlier attributed to blindness greater powers of abstraction, and deduced separately that altered sensorial conditions have effects on the reasoning processes including ethics and morality, the stage is now set to use the character of Saunderson as a philosophical mouthpiece for Diderot's materialist philosophy and potential atheism. Less engaged by the visual wondrousness of nature and its aesthetic splendours, the blind mathematician may take a step back into abstraction, the better to reason without distraction. Assigning to the blind powers of insight and a rich interiority as a result of their lack of vision is a common trope in literature. The brief autobiographical preface from Saunderson's book is soon exhausted of facts, so Diderot next refers to the seemingly authoritative work of 1747, *The Life and Character of Dr. Nicholas Saunderson, late Lucasian Professor of the Mathematics in the University of Cambridge, by his disciple and friend William Inchlif Esqr*. However, this text never existed, and Diderot's earlier marvelling at the blind man's mathematical and geometric abilities devolves into something very different. In a section of the *Lettre* that purports to describe Saunderson's deathbed confessions, a long speech from Saunderson expounds a materialist argument concerning the difficulty of believing in the existence of God for the blind.

This moment occurs in the *Lettre* rather abruptly, when Diderot explains that Saunderson, nearing death, summoned 'a clergyman of great ability' by the name of Gervase Holmes to facilitate a 'discussion on the existence of God' (1916a: 108–9). Holmes is indeed mentioned in the biographical preface to the first volume of Saunderson's *Elements of Algebra*. But Diderot's claim that fragments of the dialogue survived is pure fiction. Upon being informed by the Revd Holmes that his illness had advanced to a point beyond hope of recovery, the last words of the biographical account in the *Elements* reveal a remarkably stoical attitude:

> He received this notice of his approaching death with great calmness and serenity, and after a short silence, resumed life and spirits, and talked with as much composure of mind as he had ever done in his most sedate hours of perfect health. He appointed the evening of the following day to receive the sacrament with Mr Holmes; but before that came, he was seized with a delirium, which continued to his death. (Saunderson 1741: I, xix)

It is entirely possible that Diderot, being acquainted with this biographical detail, seized upon Saunderson's reputation for having a lack of interest in theology, along with this concrete episode of delirium in anticipation of death, to write the entirely fantastical deathbed confession, employing Saunderson as the mouthpiece for the expression of atheistic materialism. An earlier work of 1747, *Promenade du sceptique* ['The sceptic's walk'], had rehearsed some of Diderot's sceptical arguments regarding religious faith and Catholicism in particular, but the *Lettre* was able to further these views through the semi-fictionalised persona of an able and respected blind subject. 'As he lies dying, Saunderson evolves from an *empiric* – one who relies on practical and sensory experience – into a practitioner of speculative philosophy', writes Curran (2000: 89). Diderot takes up where the 'Memoirs' in the *Elements of Algebra* leaves off, presenting a deathbed conversation about the existence of God and the perception of divine order between the Revd Holmes and the delirious Saunderson. In short, Saunderson's blindness becomes a convenient device to confront the sighted vicar and voice doubt about his faith on the grounds that it relies on the wondrous spectacle of nature, a spectacle he cannot see. For a blind man like Saunderson, then, nature unfolds in an entirely random way, through blind forces, as it were:

> 'Ah, sir,' replied the blind philosopher, 'don't talk to me of this magnificent spectacle, which it has never been my lot to enjoy. I have been condemned to spend my life in darkness, and you cite wonders quite out of my understanding, and which are only evidence for you and for those who see as you do. If you want to make me believe in God you must make me touch Him'. (Diderot 1916a: 109)

Atheists, especially those with scientific inclinations, are used to accusations of a lack of wonder about the complexity of the natural world and the emergence of order within it, known as the teleological argument for God's existence or the argument from design, and generally attributed to Aquinas. If this order cannot be perceived even by an eminent mathematician, and a deity cannot be perceived except by touch, then Saunderson is fundamentally no better than the Puiseaux man, whose idea of seeing the moon at a distance was conceived in terms of long arms. Conversely, the advanced capabilities of the blind Saunderson allow Diderot to voice an alternative viewpoint about the virtues of materialism, something that is indeed tangible but without the aesthetic distractions of vision. In which case, Saunderson's reasoning abilities are able to see through arguments about the existence of God based on a visual aesthetic of divine order.

Even though there was a correspondence between Voltaire and Diderot for almost three decades, only a short exchange of letters concerned the *Lettre* specifically. This might have been because of the uncomfortable resonances of Saunderson's atheistic arguments, despite the literary devices used by the author to distance himself from them. Cru writes of this correspondence: 'The two letters of Voltaire and Diderot concerning the *Letter on the Blind* illustrate in a significant manner the parting of the ways not only between their authors, but between the two generations of French philosophers which belong to the first and second half of the eighteenth century' (1913: 169). Cru further argues that the correspondence also means a final separation between Diderot's philosophy and English deism. Locke, despite his project of a radical empiricism and interest in psychology, nevertheless remained a committed Christian throughout his life. Diderot, while voicing a materialism through the character of Saunderson, was not exactly a systematic materialist, nor was he philosophically advancing arguments about materialism or atomism much beyond Lucretius' six books of the *De rerum natura*, which goes further than most to posit a creation without a creator. Blind forces, contingencies, unstable forms, and a dynamic universe challenge any ability to impose order, even visual order, upon it. As such, the 'blind mathematician's dilemma', as Curran puts it, is insufferable: 'for him, Newton's mathematical world of perfection is untouchable and abstruse while the world open to him – the tactile and concrete world – remains unequivocally faulted' (2000: 88). Saunderson, in this case, is rendered a wretched figure, a 'passive monster' who asserts himself as living proof of another way of 'seeing' the Godless and disordered universe; in Curran's words, replacing 'divine intention' with 'blind mechanical contingencies' (2000: 89).

Diderot and the Molyneux question

Like his philosophical forebears, the importance of the Molyneux question for Diderot remains consistent with the Enlightenment interest in blindness. 'Blindness is then an absence or gap in the plenum of sense experience that enables one to know what sight is', as Creech puts it (1986: 111). The hypothetical blind man was a somewhat flimsy confection for philosophical conjecture, bearing only a shadowy relation to any actual blind man, a deficiency which Diderot fully intended to rectify, with uneven results. But the lure of the Enlightenment trope of blindness as blankness remained strong, and as Paulson argues, the *aveugle-né* remains to all intents and purposes a hypothetical naïf, such as occurs in an early developmental stage, before the multiple streams of sensory experience can combine, interweave, and provide the full sensory richness of a world with its order: 'The blind man's difference is invoked only to permit the reader's mind to perceive, as it were, a mirror of its former self, itself as it was before the accretions of conventions, judgments, and interpretive mechanisms that time and the interplay of the senses have put at its disposal' (1987: 40). This would later be a key methodological consideration for Condillac's *Traité*, of course. With all the developments since Molyneux of surgical techniques, the increased number of operations, ceremonial unbandagings, and studies of post-operative vision, and more importantly for Diderot, with the supposed benefit of extended interviews with actual blind subjects, at this point Diderot considers himself in a position to address the Molyneux problem:

> [T]he first time the eyes of one born blind open to the light, he will see nothing at all; some time will be necessary for his eye to practise sight; it will practise alone and without the aid of touch, and will eventually distinguish not only colours but the main outlines of objects. (1916a: 134)

Diderot tries to answer definitively, siding with the empiricist position since there is no mutual education of the senses wherein spatial form spontaneously arises. Likewise, the entry by d'Alembert to the *Encyclopédie* that summarises Diderot's ideas on blindness gives a nod to Voltaire's phraseology of learning to see:

> From the result of these experiments, it must clearly appear, that the sense of feeling arrives at perfection but by slow degrees, and is at first very confused; and that we learn to see, pretty nearly, as we learn to speak. A newborn babe, that opens its eyes for the first time to the light, feels, no doubt, the same progressive emotions, which have been observed in the lad born blind [i.e. Cheselden's patient]. By the agency of feeling, and custom, the erroneous judgments of infant sight are corrected gradually. (d'Alembert 1772: X, 'Aveugle')

Diderot's contribution to the long-running debate is less a philosophical framing of the problem in terms of epistemology, and more a psychological framing, given the absence of sight, concerning a shifted register of sensory attention and its bearing upon the developing nature of consciousness and the mental operations of the blind. There is, then, a specificity about blindness in terms of epistemological development and differentiation that Diderot attends to. As Paulson explains: 'By examining forms of thought and knowledge in the blind, rather than simply considering them to be deprived of visual concepts but otherwise like the seeing, Diderot implies that the nature of the senses, considered both singly and collectively, has a shaping and transforming effect on what passes through them' (1987: 55). Diderot not only opens up a significant line of inquiry in terms of how sensory epistemologies are formulated over time, but also understands that there is a difference in the discursive means by which blind subjects articulate that knowledge. There is no means by which vision could be a universal sign system that has access to, or interoperability with, other tactile or auditory signs. The blind therefore mark their difference through their four senses as opposed to the sighted's five, and so 'pose the problem of a radically different language of the senses' (Paulson 1987: 40).

Diderot asserts that the observations of the newly sighted subject will depend on the discursive capabilities furnished through the available senses by which, while still blind, they had understood their previously tactile perceptions. Having the ability to misunderstand concepts or ideas that are second nature to the sighted, with sometimes comedic effect such as mirrors or the distance to the moon, should not obscure the fact that certain abstract concepts and realms of knowledge are pursued with great acuity. As such, the dramatic moment of restoration of sight fails to reveal anything truly important, thinks Diderot.

> In no case does the moment of first sight have any special importance; it brings neither recognition of forms nor a failure to recognize. Only by comparing his new perceptions with his old ones will the subject be able to answer the question. The subject who cannot compare them will be unable to answer, and the others will answer according to their differential means of making the comparison. (Paulson 1987: 46)

This is a relatively sophisticated psychological model that not only posits a relative variance in perceptual ability and sensory discrimination, but also further implies a variance in the ability to articulate such experience, since there is no universal sensory language or sign system. To look for a single, universal truth after sight restoration may be dramatic, but is not the revelatory moment other philosophers had anticipated.

While the *aveugle-né* is able to make compensations and adjustments in terms of the recognition of objects, and after a while spatial navigation through other senses, it would be absurd to assume that the mechanisms of vision would work straight away, since even a paralysed limb must be exercised before it becomes capable once again. After sight restoration, according to Diderot, in order for the *aveugle-né* to recognise objects tactually, he must in fact have experience of both senses in order to judge, and we should not be surprised if, upon approaching a sphere and a cube, his expectations are deceived and a sphere is felt when a cube is approached, and vice versa. In other words, it is primarily a correlation built up through experience: 'Experience alone can teach me whether there be any analogy between sight and touch' (Diderot 1916a: 121). So far, this hews closely to Berkeley. With the benefit of Cheselden's report, Diderot rejects Condillac's first metaphysical explanation in *Essai sur l'origine des connaissances humaines*, later revised for *Traité des sensations*, which conceived of a psychological relation between touch and space wherein touch aids and informs the eye. Newborn infants receive light from objects at the back of the eye, which clearly does not equate with vision. But touch is indispensable in correlating and correcting those visual impressions over time:

> [C]onsequently, *we see nothing the first time we use our eyes*; and during the first moments of sight we only receive a mass of confused sensations, which are only disentangled after a time and by a process of reflection. It is by experience alone that we learn to compare our sensations with what occasions them; that sensations having no essential resemblance with their objects, it is from experience that we are to inform ourselves concerning analogies which seem to be merely positive. In short, that touch is of great service in giving the eye an accurate knowledge of the conformity of the object to the sense-impression received of it is unquestionable (1916a: 126–7, emphasis added)

The evidence put forward by Diderot about the actual experiences of blindness and space in the *Lettre* was challenged by later findings. For example, Platner in 1785 cast doubt on the veracity of Diderot's empirical information. Against Diderot's deduction that tactile experience is inherently spatial, Platner concluded after investigation that the congenitally blind literally have no awareness of space, and in the words of psychologist von Senden in *Space and Sight*, the sighted are simply 'deceived by the verbal habits of the blind' when speaking of space, since they cannot share spatial understandings with the sighted (1960: 28). Von Senden's views in turn proved controversial and were later discredited, as the spatial abilities of the blind and vision-impaired became better documented (see e.g. Degenaar 1996: 109–10). This only underlines the perspicacity of Diderot's observation that the apprehension of the object through the conformity of visual and tactile means implies a spatial component, and like exercising a formerly paralysed limb, the eye would become trained through its ongoing correlations with touch.

Towards a tactile language: de Salignac and L'Addition

Written some thirty-four years after the *Lettre* and then appended to later editions, *L'Addition à la lettre sur les aveugles* ['Addition to the preceding letter'] of 1782 is notable for almost directly contradicting points from the earlier text, and given the early apology for non-attendance at Réaumur's unbandaging event and the subsequent spirit of independent inquiry, involving interviewing the blind man from Puiseaux and the mathematician Saunderson, it seems odd that in the later work Diderot confesses to having been present at one of the many cataract operations that oculist Jacques Daviel performed (a footnote estimates an unlikely 226 in one month, November, alone). Not only does Diderot provide swathes of reported speech from some blind subjects operated upon, but a passing comment concerning one of the operations – 'I believe Marmontel and I were present on the same day' (1916b: 145) – adds a sense of first-person immediacy and authority in witnessing the event that was lacking in the *Lettre* several decades before. Another blind subject operated upon by Daviel, a blacksmith twenty-five years without sight, 'had grown so accustomed to the guidance of touch that he had to be forced to use the sense which had been restored to him. Daviel would beat him and say, "Use your eyes you wretch!" He walked, and moved, and did all that we do with our eyes open, with his eyes shut' (1916b: 144).

The blind subject most critical to *L'Addition* is the Mademoiselle Mélanie de Salignac. Diderot describes a friendship with her starting in 1760 and lasting until her death at the age of twenty-two in 1763. In 1782, aged sixty-nine, Diderot was considering editing his works and remembered the friendship with Mélanie and, according to Weygand (2009: 71), the many comments and critiques she had offered him about the *Lettre*. Initial observations about her character and the nature of her blindness in *L'Addition* are, as in the initial description of the Puiseaux man in the *Lettre*, rather general. Although blind since infancy, she was not anxious to see, she explained to Diderot, in disarmingly narcissistic terms: 'The reason [...] is that then I should only have my own eyes, whereas now I have the use of everybody's; by this loss I am always an object of loss and pity, at every instant people do me kindnesses, and at every instant I am grateful. Alas! if I could see, no one would trouble about me' (1916b: 147). Shortly afterwards, her understanding of the errors that plague vision reveals a more considered antipathy towards the possibility of seeing. Employing some limit cases for vision that nevertheless correctly express the ambiguities of the visual world as compared with the familiar certainties of touch, she offers some surprisingly perspicacious examples for a blind subject. 'I stand [...] at the entrance of a long alley; and there is a certain object at its far end. One of my friends sees it moving; another sees it stationary; one says it is an animal, another that it is a man; and on approaching it, it turns out to be a tree-stump' is one example; another illustration neatly refers us back to Voltaire's similarly ambiguous visual image that is resolved later through touch: 'No one can tell if the tower they see in the distance is round or square' (1916b: 147). Diderot noticed how, like the blind mathematician Saunderson, she showed adeptness in the abstract and calculable pursuits of astronomy, geometry, and algebra, and especially geometry since it had such universal application and no external aid or equipment was necessary. Her explanation to Diderot was succinct: 'The geometrician [...] spends nearly all his life with his eyes shut' (1916b: 152).

At one point Mélanie is probed about the visualisation techniques involved in performing her geometrical operations, and demonstrates this translatability and figuration in terms of touch. She is asked to conceive of a cube with a central point and to divide it into equal parts, and she immediately reports the division into six pyramids each with a height equal to half that of the cube. 'True,' says Diderot, 'but tell me how you see this.' She replies: 'In my head, as you do' (1916b: 153). This kind of operation is straightforward to visualise for the sighted, and perhaps for those blind with some residual vision. But in *L'Addition* Diderot attempts to grasp how such visualisation works for someone blind from infancy, and he is only able to hypothesise in terms of sensory denomination from other senses:

> I must admit I have never been able clearly to understand how she represented figures in her head without the aid of colour. Was her cube formed from memories of sensations of touch? Had her brain become, as it were, a hand within which substances were realised? Had a connection between two senses been established? Why does this connection not exist in my case, and why do I picture nothing that is not coloured in my mind's eye? What is the imagination of a blind man? This phenomenon is by no means easy of explanation. (1916b: 153)

The conscious echo of the cube and sphere from the Molyneux question, and the possibility of different senses being connected as a result, obscures the fact that Diderot is asking very different questions about blindness and the character of the imagination here. A further analogy between hands and eyes is later voiced by Mélanie when she boasts, as did Saunderson in the preceding *Lettre*, that tactile drawings on the surface of the skin would be recognised. Saunderson 'saw by means of his skin' (1916b: 107), including the traces of shapes. But Mélanie conceptualises this differently: 'My hand would become a sensitive mirror,' she opines, and she conceives the eye as a more sensitive hand, 'a living canvas of infinite delicacy' (1916b: 155) able to discern colour even. She argues through the now-familiar analogy, imagining a translation without redundancy from sight to touch: 'If the skin of my hand was as sensitive as your eye, I should see with my hand as you see with your eyes; and I sometimes imagine there are animals who have no eyes, but can nevertheless see' (1916b: 156).

If Mélanie needed no equipment for her geometrical operations because of her powers of visualisation, she nonetheless had to be adept in the use of specialised equipment for reading and writing to be proficient in other areas of learning, using elevated cut-out letters for reading and wooden frames to guide her writing, methods taught her by a tutor in much the same manner as her near-contemporary, Maria Theresia von Paradis. To what extent could such experiments in tactile writing and reading be developed into a universal system? Diderot offers suggestions in this area at various points in the *Lettre* and *L'Addition*. Decades before the competing writing systems for the blind eventually settled on a single standard, Braille, in these texts Diderot offers glimpses of alternative systems. The necessity to reach out to other senses as part of a linguistic impulse is present for Mélanie as it was for Saunderson, and at one point in *L'Addition* Diderot explains the means by which she reads and writes both music and letters through tactile signs: 'She had been taught music by notes in relief placed on raised lines on a large board. She read these notes with her hand, and played them on her instrument, and in a very short time she learnt to play the longest and most elaborate piece' (1916b: 152). Similarly, her handwriting was guided through slats on a page, where her pen would leave an indentation on the paper that could subsequently be read by her fingertips, and she could read books that were specially printed for her this way. It is slow and rather cumbersome, and 'if it is found that the expression by the common characters of writing is too slow for the sense of touch' (1916b: 89), as Diderot says in the *Lettre*, then an alternative and more abstract system must be considered. From considering tactile signs through musical notation and a form of handwriting for the blind, this explains Diderot's excitement about the more abstract and potentially universal system observed in Saunderson's arithmetic tables. Saunderson used rectilineal figures on a board, made by placing pegs at various points conjoined by string, to perform mathematical calculations. Diderot makes his case for a similarly abstract system for literacy that takes advantage of the particularities of the touch sense, as opposed to the available piecemeal systems or the use of standard raised letters taught only by virtue of convention. In other words, he offers the radical suggestion of a replete tactile language that would be of use in communicating not only with the blind, but also with the deaf and the mute:

> But units pure and simple are too vague and general symbols for us. Our senses bring us back to symbols more suited to our comprehension and the conformation of our organs. We have arranged that these signs should be common property and serve, as it were, for the staple in the exchange of our ideas. We have made them for our eyes in the alphabet, and for our ears in articulate sounds; but we have none for the sense of touch, although there is a way of speaking to this sense and of obtaining its responses. For lack of this language, there is no communication between us and those born deaf, blind, and mute. They grow, but they remain in a condition of mental imbecility. Perhaps they would have ideas, if we were to communicate with them in a definite and uniform manner from their infancy; for instance, if we were to trace on their hands the same letters we trace on paper, and associated always the same meaning with them. (1916b: 89)

Having a pre-formed set of tactile signs would be an immeasurable benefit, rather than having to invent them *ab initio*. But the concept is left floating, without being developed more fully. Diderot then returns to a discussion of Saunderson's mathematical system.

Conclusion: sightlessness, senses, and signs

Just as there are two modes in English that denote the lack of vision, the more metaphorical 'blindness' and the more clinical 'sightlessness', the same is true in French. The literal or medical sense of blindness that we call sightlessness, vision loss, or vision impairment is *cecité* in French, in use from the thirteenth century and deriving from the Latin *caecitas*, meaning blindness or darkness. The second, more metaphorical mode, comparable in English to speaking of 'blind faith' or being 'blind' to the truth of something, is *aveuglement*, from Old French *avogle*, which derives from the Latin *ab oculis* and was in use from the eleventh century. There is a sense in which the blind subject of Molyneux's question has been literally sightless, their blindness being *cecité*, and the epistemological question clearly deals with the hypothetical and actual restoration of sight through cataract surgery. Conversely, much of both Diderot's *Lettre* and *L'Addition* has thematically danced around more metaphorical forms of blindness, including the inability to grasp areas such as theology, metaphysics, and the spectacle of a divine order wherein all phenomena and creatures have their place. Where was the resting place for the bed-bound, delirious Saunderson, the Godless sufferer unable to conceive of, never mind actually visually perceive, the grand spectacle of nature? Based on the etymology of both *cecité* and *aveuglement*, the polarity seems reversed. *Caecitas* should work more metaphorically in terms of a persistent trope in thinking about blindness as perpetual darkness, whereas the literalness of being *ab oculis* – without eyes – should speak directly to the physiological condition of sightlessness. Years after the *Lettre*, d'Alembert, Diderot's collaborator in the famous multi-volume *Encyclopédie* compiled between 1751 and 1772, wrote an entry on 'Aveugle' ['Blind'] that revisited some of Diderot's material, recounting certain episodes about the *aveugle-né* of Puiseaux with his cane and Saunderson with his mathematical tables, but also offered a more explicit argument for the separation of the literal and metaphorical senses of blindness. The entry attempts to enforce a distinction between *cecité* and *aveuglement*, and a footnote in Curran's article explains: 'Diderot's representation of this double blindness – a concurrent physical and ethical cécité – simply combines the early modern era's use of the term «aveuglement» in both literal and figurative senses.' Curran continues: '«Aveuglement», recommends the article's author, d'Alembert, should be used figuratively in moral matters, while «cécité» should be used to describe the physical condition of sightlessness' (2000: 83 n. 13). Indeed, both the *Lettre* and *L'Addition* offer a departure from the strict ocular condition of sightlessness or recovery of sight that the Molyneux question had enshrined, and provide a more discursive treatment of the experiences and psychological conditions of 'blindness' in its wider senses.

From Voltaire and Condillac we saw developments around the senses and signs, and here through Diderot we have glimpsed a more fully articulated relationship between the senses and the spaces of representation such that a more systematic tactile language might occur. In the following chapters, we chart the subsequent systematisation and adoption of one such tactile language, Braille, and the way in which technologies of sensory substitution since the 1950s have explored and practically experimented with the spatiality of the senses and the blind sensorium. Examples and analysis of such technologies reveal the legacy not only of the Molyneux question, but also Diderot's specifically tactile language. Therefore cross-modal transfer of sensory information is at the heart of reading Braille with the fingers as well as more technologically inclined tactile-visual sensory substitution systems (TVSS), as we shall see.

Chapter 6

Reading with the Fingers: Tactile Signs and the Possibilities for a Language of Touch

The long road to literacy for the blind includes Diderot's invocation for a 'clear and precise language of touch' (1916a: 90). In the century between the *Lettre sur les aveugles* of 1749 and the official adoption of Braille in France in 1854, previous attempts at raised script were consolidated, and a fateful meeting took place in 1784 between a blind musical prodigy named Maria Theresia von Paradis and Valentin Haüy, a talented linguist and avid reader of Diderot. During this period the role of the senses in education was the subject of much interest, and the rise of sensationism in France derived from Locke by Diderot and Voltaire, and more systematically by Condillac, would have very real consequences in the first nationally recognised schools for the blind and the deaf in France. The accidental discovery in 1786 by Valentin Haüy that embossed script could be read by the fingers, for example, implied in the words of Farrell that 'sensitive fingers [...] could take the place of insensitive eyes' (1956: 93). The substitution of touch for sight, of hands for eyes, lay at the heart of the development of education for the blind. Or, in the words of Merry in an article appropriately titled 'Fingers for eyes', 'There seems always to have been among civilized people at least a vague realization that the finger should serve as the eye of the blind' (Merry 1937: 237).

In the *Lettre*, Diderot had questioned 'a sensible blind man' in order to 'understand his psychology' (1916a: 116–17), thereby subjecting him to philosophical speculations on the role of the sensorial in the elaboration of human knowledge. To be sure, sensibility was the foundation for any knowledge of the outside world and, as transpired through his interviews with blind subjects, Diderot was interested in exploring the way that sensibility also informed moral sentiment, theological questions, and even civic engagement. His recommendation of a tactile language for communication with the blind, deaf, and mute was considered not only a matter of universal ease for expression and understanding between individuals, but would also enhance the mental operations of these sensorily compromised subjects. Following Locke's famous analogy within empiricist philosophy of the blank slate, whereby knowledge is never innate and accumulated only through experience, Jennifer Riskin considers this epistemological mechanism in more social terms. If, using Locke's prevailing analogy, the Enlightenment individual began life as a blank slate, would the society of others not leave beneficial impressions upon them? As Riskin summarises: 'Experimental and philosophical writers on blindness increasingly turned to the problem of sociability and its basis in sensibility, and their preoccupation had lasting institutional effects' (2002: 22). These effects included the programmes for civic education that began to appear towards the end of the eighteenth century, and the first school for the blind in the 1780s. This school initially faced significant challenges in being recognised and established as an institution, yet within a decade it had become 'a Revolutionary symbol of the brotherly love and community that could arise from a national program of moral education' (Riskin 2002: 22).

From the initial hypothetical considerations of blindness by Locke and his popularity in France, the subsequent deliberations on the Molyneux problem and Cheselden's patient by the *philosophes* which introduced a moral dimension, and the wish on the part of experimental pedagogues to bridge solipsistic concerns with more social ones emerges a narrative of the institutional recognition of the blind. This happened, first, through a campaign by Haüy and others for the establishment of the first school for the blind in France, and secondly, through the development within that school of a tactile writing system such as Diderot had presaged, which was finally accomplished with the help of Braille in 1854. This chapter encompasses the Enlightenment themes of sensibility and the moral order, the establishment of sponsored institutions for the deaf and deafmute by the Abbé de l'Epée in 1760, and for the blind by Haüy in 1784, and the experiments with tactile writing systems in the blind school up until the official adoption of Braille. No longer the realm of idle philosophical speculations, there were now very real implications for learning, and for access to, the more abstract pursuits of literature and culture for the blind.

On sensation and education: Mérian

Between 1770 and 1780 Jean-Bernard Mérian presented a series of papers to the Berlin Academy in which he systematically detailed responses to the Molyneux problem up to that time, and analysed their underlying presuppositions. These included Leibniz's solution, written in 1704 but posthumously published only a few years previously, in 1765. Mérian was a philosopher, and along with a volume chronicling the Molyneux problem and its answers, published as *Nouveaux memoires de l'Academie Royal des Sciences et Belles-Lettres de Berlin* (1772), he also outlined an educational programme inspired by Cheselden's experiment with sight restoration in 1728 and Condillac's renowned 1754 thought experiment of the statue that progressively comes to life through the addition of each of the senses. The ideal schooling, Mérian reasoned, would similarly attend to each of the five senses independently and successively, so that none would interfere with the development of another. As we saw, Leibniz had maintained that innate ideas were present but rather confused, so the successive ordering of knowledge from each sense could only strengthen the learning process. Of course, this was impracticable, so Mérian suggested a more modest, but no less pragmatic, system in its stead: 'to take children from the cradle, and raise them in profound darkness until the age of reason', in the meantime learning through a form of raised print 'the Sciences, Physics, Philosophy, Geometry and Optics above all' (Mérian 1778, in Riskin 2002: 62 n. 122). Their minds being so cultivated, as Mérian would have it, they would emerge as fully developed rational beings into the light. A more perfect emblem of Enlightenment education and the supposed abstracted knowledge within darkness, and therefore blindness, would be difficult to find. And rather than the single blind subject of philosophical inquiry featured in Molyneux's question, Cheselden's patient, and Diderot's interview in Puiseaux, Mérian's proposal involved performing comparatively modern psychological experiments upon a whole classroom of subjects, measuring the effects of varying degrees of deprivation and education. Mérian elaborates: 'as their minds would be, so to speak, in our hands, and as we could shape them like soft wax, and develop understanding in them in whatever order we pleased, we would be in a position to take all precautions, and to vary the experiments in all imaginable ways' (in Paulson 1987: 217–18 n. 49). The malleability of the subjects' minds, effectuated through sensory deprivation, could only be a gift to an educator who desired to imprint, shape, or mould their students in decisive and dramatic ways like blank slates. Given that the bulk of their childhood would be spent sensorily deprived and artificially blind, this would heighten the moment of revelation, echoing the Enlightenment motif that Foucault identified of the blind subject seeing the world for the first time, in truth and glory:

> With what a torrent of delights will they be flooded, what will be their movements of joy, when they shall be brought from night to day, from shadows to light, when a new universe, an absolutely brilliant world, will come forth for them as from the womb of Chaos? Is there anything comparable to such a moment? (Mérian, in Paulson 1987: 218 n. 52)

If this eccentric scheme might be considered the logical culmination of previously discussed philosophical thought experiments concerning the senses, even the darkness of sensory deprivation, a more benign vision of education was being developed specifically for the blind and the deaf, involving a more socially inclusive ideal of institutions based on educational advancement and the restoration of dignity for the blind, deaf, and deaf-mute. What follows is an account of the formation of the far more pragmatically oriented, state-recognised and sponsored Institution Royale des Jeunes Aveugles, the Royal School for the Blind in Paris. This was founded by Haüy, who followed a model of education established for the deaf and deaf-mute by a contemporary, the Abbé de l'Epée, which sought to enhance literacy for the blind and aid communication through systems of tactile signs. The Abbé, whose school for the deaf and deaf-mute was founded in 1755, was still enacting a philosophy of the senses, though distinctly divergent from Mérian's. The Abbé and Haüy adopted a non-Berkeleyan view, no doubt influenced by Diderot's discussion of blind subjects learning through tactile abstractions in the *Lettre*, that the senses were parallel conduits through which knowledge entered the soul, and therefore that sensory impairments were simply the lack of one conduit among other, equally capable, senses. In other words, it was postulated that certain senses could effectively replace the functions of another sense. The Abbé had written that teaching the deaf was a matter of 'sending through their eyes into their mind what enters ours by our ears' (1784, in Riskin 2002: 63); Haüy recognised the significance of this idea, of 'impressing the soul with new ideas, in speaking to the eyes alone' and, in a letter to the *Journal de Paris* of that year, he chronicled the blind school's foundation and early history, expressing a view comparable to the Abbé's that his own students would 'replace sight by touch' (Haüy 1786, in Riskin 2002: 63).

A few years prior to Mérian's idiosyncratic excursions in pedagogy, Book II of Rousseau's *Émile, or On Education* (1762) likewise pondered the role of the senses in the instruction and education of the child: 'We are not masters of the use of all our senses equally. There is one of them – touch – whose activity is never suspended during waking. It has been spread over the entire surface of our body as a continual guard to warn us of all that can do it damage' (1979: 96). Due to its continual presence and constant use by virtue of our being embodied, and whether we are aware of it or not, touch has a life of its own and needs no special training or attention, says Rousseau. Furthermore, he repeats the assumption that the sense of touch is heightened in the blind:

> We observe that the blind have a surer and keener touch than we do; because, not being guided by sight, they are forced to learn to draw solely from the former sense the judgment which the latter furnishes us. Why, then, are we not given practice at walking as the blind do in darkness, to know the bodies we may happen to come upon, to judge the objects which surround us – in a word, to do at night without light all that they do by day without eyes? As long as the sun shines, we have the advantage over them. In the dark they are in turn our guides. We are blind half of our lives, with the difference that the truly blind always know how to conduct themselves, while we dare not take a step in the heart of the night... As for me, I prefer that Emile have eyes in the tips of his fingers than in a candle-maker's shop. (Rousseau 1979: 97)

Because of their more finely developed sense of touch, therefore, the blind are elevated to the status of teachers of the sighted, for they are at an advantage in the dark. Furthermore, touch as a sense of immediacy and proximity was better suited to communication in terms of reading and writing, and allowed blind subjects to read to themselves without the help of other people. Weygand identifies this increasing aptitude for reading and writing, for blind and sighted alike, with the increasing taste for privacy and for the practice of reading silently (2009: 69). For the blind to benefit from such literacy, whether for the purposes of educational instruction or for more private matters, required concentration on more necessarily tactile forms of reading and writing, which happened to coincide with the renewed status of touch and touching for philosophy in the wake of the Molyneux problem.

Of sensibility, sociability, and substitution: Valentin Haüy

The divergent approaches of Mérien and of de l'Epée and Haüy are symptomatic of the divide between the abstruse epistemological debate that had continued since Molyneux's original question, along with its subsequent philosophical commentaries, and the pragmatic development of a distinctly tactile language after Diderot's *Lettre*, with its potential for education, training, and actively improving the lives of the blind. Valentin Haüy, a passionate linguist who translated Italian, Spanish, and Portuguese for Louis XVI, and an expert in writing systems, had been impressed with Diderot's *Lettre*. But he developed a more pragmatic pedagogic trajectory after meeting the celebrated blind Austrian pianist and prodigy Maria Theresia von Paradis, when she was residing in Paris. Von Paradis was celebrated not only for her musical proficiency and well-developed musical memory, but also for her extensive knowledge of geography and arithmetic achieved through her specially printed tactile books and maps. In an age when innumerable obstacles stood in the way of education and inclusion for the blind, the ability to access such material, to acquire musical proficiency and knowledge of the entire world through her fingertips, was singular. Haüy was understandably keen to interview her about her use of tactile reading systems, and his own tactile teaching techniques were based on this information. If Voltaire and Condillac, following Locke, had initially sought to understand the mechanisms for knowledge through an impressionable mind, their countrymen were now concerned with how such an impressionable mind might be civilised, educated, and know its place in the wider social world. For the blind, this meant an escape from impecuniousness and the indignity of begging, to cultivate employable skills, and ultimately to rejoin literate culture, an ability that von Paradis publicly demonstrated.

For the majority of the unfortunate blind who, for whatever reason, were unable to undergo corrective surgery, an opportunity would become available that would allow them to 'escape their humiliating circumstances' (Weygand 2009: 7) through education by means of tactile reading of specially printed books with embossed signs. However, the trajectory between the acknowledgement of the possibilities of a purely tactile language and the adoption of one tactile reading system above all as a gateway to a world of literary culture and knowledge was far from straightforward. For Haüy initially had more modest, but realistic, aims. He wished for his blind subjects to read and write as an escape from the misery of grinding poverty, to enhance their effectiveness in the workplace, 'to employ those among them who are in easy circumstances in an agreeable manner', and more generally 'to render useful to society their hands' (1894: 10). The pedagogical possibilities of forms of substitution of one sense for another had been raised by figures such as Rousseau and Mérian, as we saw. According to this view, if the senses were indeed conduits, then blindness merely involved an obstruction in one of several perfectly functional sources of potential knowledge, and some form of redress could be made accordingly. Here, argues Riskin, was 'the central axiom of Haüy's pedagogy' (2002: 63). As the talented blind prodigies had shown, the blind need not be reduced to imbecility, and the potential for education through the remaining senses could be great.

Innovations in printing techniques, some of which von Paradis would demonstrate to Haüy at their meeting, would accordingly use the sense of touch to open the minds, if not the eyes, of the blind to a whole world outside of their solitary darkness. As Haüy enthused in his *Essai sur l'education des aveugles* ['Essay on the education of the blind'] (1786), these new technologies of raised printing would provide some necessary momentum to transform the lives of the blind through an education based on touch. 'Let them only, by means of reading', he proposed in his *Essai*, find a remedy 'against that intolerable melancholy, which corporeal darkness, and mental inactivity' made their habitual state (1894: 15). The same connection between the senses and social membership, of opening up the social world through touch, was also stressed by the Academie Royal des Sciences et Belles-Lettres, which thereby formally approved Haüy's mission. Haüy's pedagogical approach through touch not only gave the blind 'knowledge that the deprivation of the most necessary sense has refused them', but also would 'open them ... to the society of other men' (Académie des Sciences 1785, in Riskin 2002: 64). To be accepted into the society of other men, as the Académie would have it, meant to be folded back into the world of literacy and learning, on the one hand, but also moral rectitude, a return to the concerns of society in all its facets and functions. In this way, recovering the blind, as also the deaf and deaf-mute, from a state of moral isolation was a driving factor in gaining recognition from the state and the Académie for blind education.

In this sense the school was emblematic, and advertised its progressive direction to the public through a series of public displays. Haüy's school 'was a living symbol, to which the enlightened and fashionable came in throngs every Wednesday and Friday to witness the blind students' "public exercises"' (Riskin 2002: 66). Clearly, literacy was a key factor in communicating ideas to the blind, and this Haüy wished to address. His *Essai* summarised his new purpose: 'to teach the blind reading, by the assistance of books, where the letters are rendered palpable by their elevation above the surface of the paper and by means of this reading, to instruct them in the art of printing, of writing, of arithmetic, the languages, history, geography, mathematics and music, &c.' (1894: 10). However, what Haüy imagined would be read was limited in scope at first to educational materials which would make the blind useful and productive, to train them for mechanical operations to aid their employment in spinning, weaving, and bookbinding, rather than fully embracing the abstract pleasures of literary culture as such. That would come in time.

An incident at the blind café

A few decades after Diderot's *Lettre*, Haüy's experience at the so-called 'Café des Aveugles' in 1771 initiated efforts to raise the blind out of their humiliating circumstances and allow them to aspire to, and have increased access to, means of self-improvement through literacy. There was a striking parallel at this time with the teaching of the deaf. The recognition of the deaf and the blind in Paris, and the acknowledgement of the necessity for literacy, were championed separately but concurrently by two different figures, but with similar aims and results. The Abbé Charles-Michel de L'Epée had devoted his life to the poor in the slums of Paris, and there he had observed two deaf sisters communicating through signs. He set up a school in 1760 to teach a group of deaf-mutes using what he would call a 'language of methodical signs' (Seigel 1995: 107ff.), believing that in this way they would be able to receive the sacraments. In a mode that would become familiar from those advocating the education and rights of the blind at the time, he explains the language of methodical signs in terms of sensory substitution: 'the education of deaf mutes must teach them through the eye what other people acquire through the ear' (in Lebars 1913: 484). The Abbé and his school played a singular role in advocating the plight of the deaf to the public and gaining recognition for their rights, and having been renamed several times the school remains as the Institut National de Jeunes Sourds de Paris (National Institute of Deaf Youth). We saw how Diderot's *Lettre sur les sourds et muets* was initially and falsely premised on a hypothesis of an entirely natural system of gestures, a view evidently shared by the Abbé. In 1771 the Abbé presented deaf-mute students from the school to the public for the first time, effectively demonstrating the viability of this means of systematic communication. An early incarnation of sign language, it soon outgrew the Abbé's initial religious intentions, becoming a fully fledged sign system and medium of expression for the deaf for all manner of subjects, although abstract concepts were cumbersome and unintuitive to sign.

Several versions exist of the experience that Haüy supposedly underwent in 1771, the same year as the Abbé's public performance of deaf-mutes communicating through signing. At one point in his *Essai*, Haüy summarises the episode at the Café des Aveugles and describes it as formative not only of his attitude to the blind, but also as a stimulus for considering the role of education in improving their lives, and the centrality of literacy in this. As a result, this episode has haphazardly entered into a larger mythology of blindness, being repeated in articles and books for blind and sighted alike, for example De La Sizeranne's book *The Blind as Seen Through Blind Eyes* (1894), originally published in French in 1889; Sir Francis J. Campbell's entry 'Blindness' in the 1910 edition of the *Encyclopaedia Britannica*; and Koestler's history of blindness in the United States, *The Unseen Minority*, originally published in 1976. During St Ovid's Fair, Haüy visited the kind of café where respectable citizens socialise after work. It must have been startling to see a group of people from the Quinze-Vingts hospice in Paris performing for the amusement of the sighted public. 'Eight or ten blind persons, with spectacles on their noses, placed along a desk which sustained instruments of music, where they executed a discordant symphony, seemed to give delight to the audience.' Of course, Haüy had a dissimilar reaction to that of the audience, and in the dumbshow of mock music reading he found an insight into the possibilities for actual literacy for the blind:

> Seated on a high platform outside a café in what is now the Place Vendôme were a handful of blind men scraping away discordantly at an assortment of musical instruments. On their noses hung huge empty pasteboard spectacles; to emphasize their blindness, the inscribed sides of the candlelit music scores faced away from them. As though this were not ridicule enough, the men were costumed in grotesque robes and crowned with dunce caps adorned with asses' ears. An advertising poster caricatured the scene to attract customers to the Café des Aveugles. (Koestler 1976: 397)

Koestler's account of this episode perhaps heightens for dramatic effect both Haüy's outrage and the indignity of the actual spectacle, where the blind men are described as grotesquely costumed, clowning around, and mimicking the actions of the sighted. With enormous false spectacles placed on their noses, their performance included a childlike parody of the act of reading. What the public found unreservedly hilarious – the grotesque parody of acts of seeing, heightened to absurdity through comic props and over-the-top movements – filled Haüy's heart instead with profound disquiet. Within this grotesque display, we might say, the 'monstration' was evident, and the willingness of the blind to participate in their bizarre pantomime disappointed him. According to Weygand's translation he considered this 'a dishonor to the human race' (2009: 7), and Koestler translates Haüy's words as an 'outrage to humanity' (1976: 397). From this moment Haüy vowed to enable the blind to read in actuality, not as a mocking display, and resolved to see his name remembered for the creation of a universal language for the blind: 'I will make the blind to read! I will put in their hands volumes printed by themselves. They will trace the true characters and will read their own writing, and they shall be enabled to execute harmonious concerts' (Haüy, in Koestler 1976: 397).

Despite his dismay, Haüy allowed himself more sober reflection on the experience at the Café des Aveugles in his *Essai*, and considered some practical implications for the blind performers:

> A very different sentiment possessed our soul, and we conceived, at that very instant, the possibility of realizing, to the advantage of those unfortunate people, the means of which they had only an apparent and ridiculous enjoyment: the blind, said we to ourselves, do they not know objects by the diversity of their forms? Are they mistaken in the value of a piece of money? Why can they not distinguish a C from G in music, or an *a* from an *f* in orthography, if their characters were rendered plain? (1894: 30)

Whether or not the performers in this case could actually play their instruments, it was becoming apparent that some virtuoso musicians and child prodigies were touring Europe and impressing audiences despite the challenge and stigma of being blind. One such celebrated blind musician was Maria Theresia von Paradis. Celebrated or not, the necessity for any blind person to distinguish letters correctly and to read without orthographic error meant that Haüy needed to acquaint himself with the advantages or shortcomings of whichever tactile writing systems were then available. His vision that volumes would be printed by the blind themselves would take over ten years to achieve, and was precipitated by a meeting with von Paradis after one of her fêted performances in Paris.

Experiments in tactile writing

From the meeting between von Paradis and Haüy it was clear that prior attempts at printing and writing by the blind were unsystematic but replete with potential. Wolfgang von Kempelen, renowned for his mechanical inventions, including most famously the chess-playing automaton known as the Mechanical Turk (see Standage 2002 for an excellent account), had taught von Paradis to read using cardboard letters, and furnished her with a small writing device consisting of a manual press which allowed her to print letters to her many correspondents. Another tutor, Niesen, had developed a system of brass letters that he passed down to his student Wiessenberg, who in turn offered von Paradis this equipment along with tactile playing cards and calculating tables, based on designs by the blind mathematician Saunderson. So when von Paradis met Haüy in Paris and showed specially printed 'geographical maps, playing cards, arithmetic tables' (Weygand 2009: 75), these had been passed down through a privileged system of blind tutelage. She showed him a printed letter, probably from Weissenburg's machine, that was full of delicate and well-expressed sentiments. Haüy was struck by this more artful use of the tactile medium: 'This attempt gave birth in my mind to the idea of applying the blind to the art of printing for the use of those who see' (1894: 20). Bernouilli had taught a young blind girl to write, and Weissenburg who himself was blind from the age of seven had devised a writing machine, and these precedents encouraged Haüy to teach his own blind students to write. Weissenburg had used a pointed instrument to inscribe letters *in relievo*, but Haüy pioneered a system of placing a frame on to the paper that separates into several horizontal lines to guide the writer's hand. From this could be developed a printing system where metal block type could be inserted for printing, and even figures for performing arithmetic calculations, following from the blind mathematician Saunderson's system.

Thirteen years after the episode at St Ovid's Fair, and inspired by his recent meeting with von Paradis, a chance encounter with a young blind man presented Haüy with an opportunity to subject a blind subject to experiments in tactile writing. A seventeen-year-old boy named François Le Sueur, blind since the age of six weeks, was found begging on behalf of his parents at the church of Saint-Germain des Prés (Haüy 1894: 31). There was now increased public awareness of certain outstanding blind prodigies, such as Saunderson in England and Weissenburg in Germany, and Haüy saw potential in taking in Le Sueur as a student. Donations were secured, and he showed an inclination to study. Haüy experimented with various tactile forms of reading including, first, raised moveable type arranged between horizontal grooves on a board and, secondly, perforations in paper made by a pin. Describing these experiments, Haüy declared: 'Already had the wonders of the art of writing, which before had appeared chimerical, been realized. Already, under their touch, which was now found a substitute for vision, had the conceptions of the blind assumed a body' (1894: 12). These elementary but workable forms of reading, along with Le Sueur's demonstration of his enthusiasm for study, impressed a group of influential visitors including the magistrate, an aptly named Monsieur Le Noir (1894: 32). As a result the Philanthropic Society provided for the assistance of twelve blind children, and thus arose the first blind school. On 19 February 1786 the Royal Academy of Music in Paris performed a concert for the blind students, and members of the public were given a demonstration of their study skills, including reading and mathematics. Whether Haüy felt uncomfortable echoes of that display of mock learning at the Café des Aveugles thirteen years earlier was not recorded. However, the sagacity of engaging officials and a well-meaning public to believe, along with him, in the virtues of encouraging literacy and learning in the blind meant that the school was on a strong footing. By the time Haüy wrote the *Essai* later that year the school had doubled in size, from thirteen students to thirty.

The next development in tactile literacy came from an accidental discovery. Le Sueur was tidying his teacher's papers and found an invitation card with heavily embossed characters. A letter 'O' was readily tangible. In a state of excitement the boy showed Haüy that he could decipher several other letters, and Haüy immediately carved other letters into the card with a knife which were, in turn, recognised. The realisation that embossing characters on paper was a workable solution to literacy opened the door to a world of learning and scholarship. To proceed, leaves of books were assembled with embossed italic characters, glued in pairs so that both the front and back of each page were readable by the blind students. Obviously this made each embossed book comparatively thicker and heavier than its normally printed counterpart, with increased demands on library storage. But an advantage of this embossed method was that the same printing press could be used, with only minor modifications, to produce either raised letter or the traditional ink transfer printing:

> We ordered typographical characters to be cast of the form in which their impression strikes our eyes, and by applying to these a paper wet, as the printers do, we produced the first exemplar which had till then appeared of letters whose elevation renders them obvious to the touch without the intervention of sight. Such was the origin of a library for the use of the blind. (Haüy 1894: 12)

Further refinement of the embossing process involved variations in the size of script, and modifying the metal printing plate so that, instead of having a hard metal or wood surface, it had a layer of a soft, rubber-like material. Thus, when clamped down on the type, the softer surface allowed the shapes of the lead type to emboss the paper. As the process was refined and the quality of rubber improved, raised letter printing became more commonplace. As Merry observes, these experiments in printing made the assumption, first, that the blind must be educated through identical means to the sighted, except through the tactile medium; and secondly, that there was a positive relationship between size and tangibility, such that the larger the script the easier it was to read. Both assumptions proved erroneous (Merry 1937: 274). The readability of tactile signs would depend on other factors, eventually breaking with any necessity for verisimilitude between tactile pattern and visual letter, and scaling the tactile pattern to best suit those parts of the fingers with the greatest tactile acuity, the fingertips. It would be seventy years until the break with visual letters was complete.

In the meantime, increased tactile acuity helped the blind reader discern patterns even if they smoothed out after use, noted Haüy (1894: 14). The mechanism of cylindrical printing *in relievo* allowed different kinds of tactile surfaces to be produced for the blind, including 'musical characters, geographical maps, the principal strokes of designing [blueprints and plans], and, in general, of all the figures of which the knowledge may be obtained by means of touch' (Haüy 1894: 19). Haüy's enthusiasm for communicating diverse knowledge through touch was no doubt precipitated by the meeting with von Paradis and her demonstrations of von Kempelen's and Wiessenberg's writing machines. Through such *in relievo* printing techniques stocks of knowledge were built up through libraries of tactile materials, 'rendering printing useful to the blind for their own use' (Haüy 1894: 20). But the vision of standardising tactile printing techniques lay not only in the reading and comprehension of ideas from the sighted world by the blind, but also in a more symmetrical arrangement whereby blind artists and writers could communicate to their sighted audience.

As more blind institutions became established in France, England, and around the world, more printing presses were adapted to further this method of literacy for the blind. The first book to be printed with embossed letters in the United States came out in Philadelphia in 1833, using a modification of the Roman alphabet to enhance tangibility (Merry 1937: 274). In Germany a modification to the embossed print outlined the text through a serrated form, enhancing the tangibility and to some extent prefiguring Braille. The New England Institution for the Education of the Blind in Boston under the direction of Samuel

Gridley Howe, later to become the Perkins Institute, obtained its first printing press in 1835, and began publishing several works in a tactile format. By 1842 it had produced the New Testament, the complete text of the Bible, a universal history, as well as geography, grammar, and spelling books. Having appraised a number of available embossed writing scripts, Howe introduced one that would become known as Boston line letter. Reading long sentences was burdensome, however, and the mastering of reading through tactile means was laborious and time-consuming, irrespective of enthusiastic public displays of blind reading and learning for funding purposes. Unsurprisingly therefore, a more systematic and efficient means of printing and reading for the blind was in development, and while its adoption was initially slow, a novel form of tactile-spatial arrangement would eventually become the universal standard in literacy for the blind.

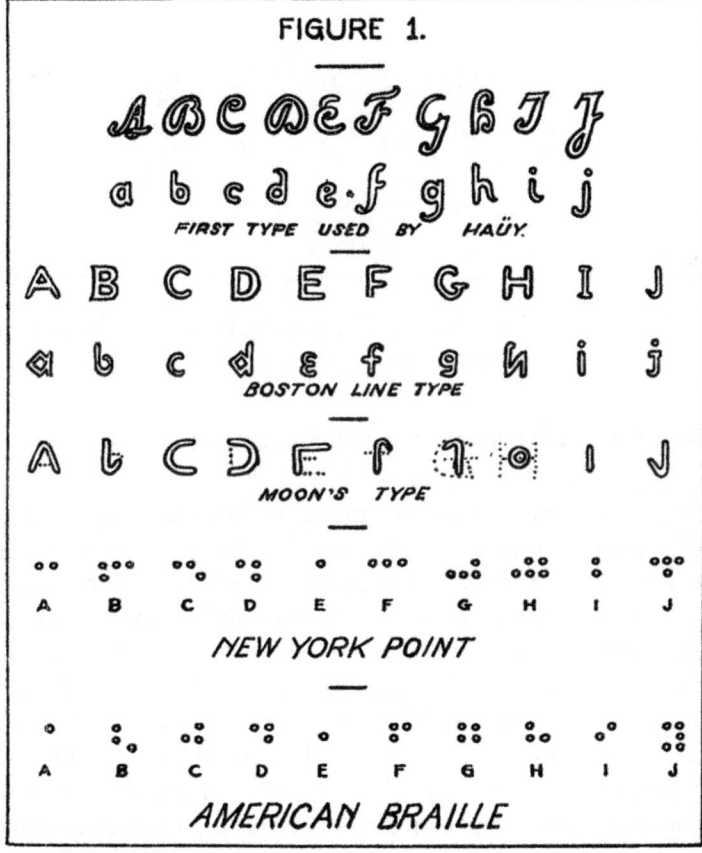

Figure 6.1 An illustration of competing tactile writing systems. From Merry (1937), 'Fingers for eyes', p. 275.

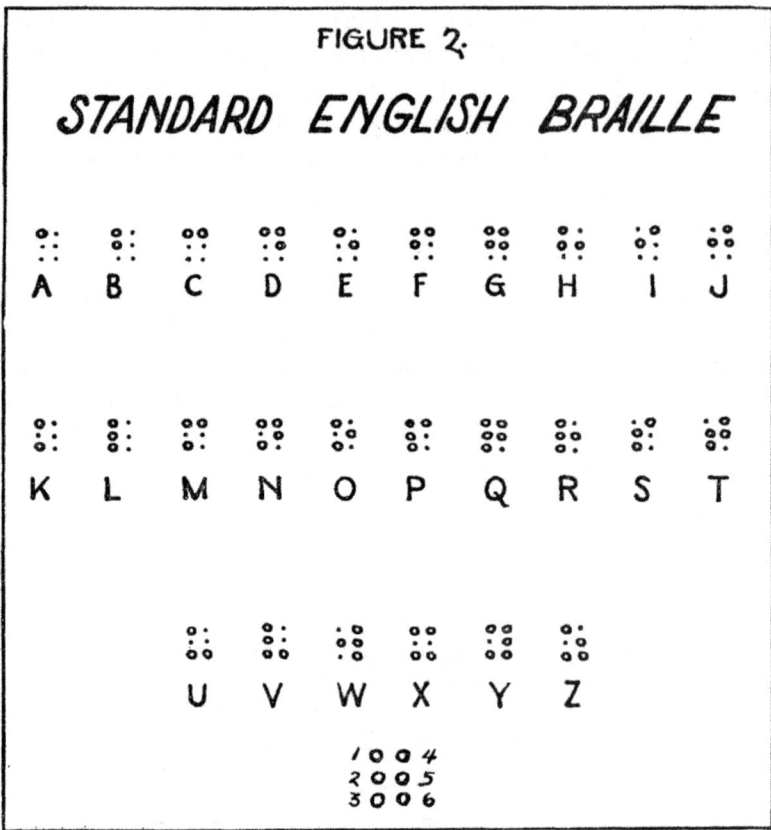

Figure 6.2 Standard English Braille, illustration from Merry (1937), 'Fingers for eyes', p. 276.

Reading, abstraction, and distraction

Given their customary social and moral isolation, Haüy believed that the blind suffered from a reduced sensibility. In the absence of the musical gifts or talents of such a one as Maria Theresia von Paradis, left to their own devices the blind intellect would become dull. Diderot had identified a tendency towards abstraction, a tendency personified in Saunderson's tactile calculating tables. An avid reader of Diderot and Rousseau, it was no stretch for Haüy to remark on the 'astonishing' talent for abstract mental operations that the blind exhibited, stating it as well known 'what a clear conception the greatest number of them discover in the difficult operations of the mind', abilities that included 'so great a propensity for calculation that we have often seen them following an arithmetical process, and correcting its errors, by memory alone' (Haüy 1894: 23). D'Alembert had made a similar claim in his *Encyclopédie* entry on 'Blindness', the blind being able to concentrate their minds without the endless procession of visual distractions that blight the sighted or, in Haüy's words, 'the crowd of images the impressions of which cross ceaselessly through our brain despite us' (Haüy, in Riskin 2002: 65). The lack of such distraction permitted a more calming darkness that was conducive to study. In other words, there was nothing to counter the generally held assumption, present in Diderot but repeated in philanthropic writing at the time, that the blind were naturally abstract thinkers. This assumption would continue unchallenged into the nineteenth century, the director of the Institut des Jeunes Aveugles, de Guillié, writing categorically in 1817 that the blind 'see things in a more abstract manner than we do' (in Paulson 1987: 112). Yet despite such simplistic assumptions, could this not partly constitute an argument about blind literacy through the translatability from touch to sight? Weissenburg's writing machine, Saunderson's calculating tables, the tactile maps and charts circulated to other generations of blind students like von Paradis – did they not assume a capacity for abstraction such that collections of tactile marks, signs, and symbols were read sequentially but were capable of producing far more complex intellectual operations, such as the establishment of numerical relationships, or speculative philosophical inquiry? And was the translatability of touch for sight at the heart of this? For the coding and decoding of tactile signs, and the propensity for abstract qualities of geometric order and rhythm, are involved in the recognition of embossed letters and figures, but especially so in terms of the cognitive efficiencies and the tactile-spatial nature of the raised dot patterns of Braille, as we now investigate.

'Night writing': a new configuration of tactile signs

There were early sporadic attempts to produce a system to enable the blind to read and write by figures such as Cardano in the 1550s, Rampazetto in 1575, and Peter Moreau in Paris a century later. Rather than the haphazard system of tactile tutelage among blind teachers and students, the need to systematise a tactile writing system began to meet with the necessary innovations in printing mechanisms much later. Around the time Haüy was exploring pathways to literacy for the blind, a Monsieur Fournier in Paris in 1783 apparently 'cut punches and struck matrices in which type were cast and printed from', according to an essay of 1869 (in Oliphant 2008: 71).

The procedure was funded by M. Rouillé de l'Etrang, treasurer of the Philanthropic Society in Paris, who was instrumental in the establishment of the Institut Royale des Jeunes Aveugles. However, the path to the acceptance of a common, universal tactile language was not straightforward. Barbier's initial offer to share his system of *ecriture nocturne* or 'night writing', a system of raised symbols on a surface used by night artillery, was summarily rejected by the Institute's founder and director, de Guillié. Nevertheless, Barbier persisted and remained convinced that his system was useful for the blind (Paulson 1987: 109). Fortunately, the next director of the Institute between 1821 and 1840, Alexandre René Pignier, wished to set a more magnanimous and humanistic example for his blind students by cultivating religion and music. The change in regime between directors was marked; de Guillié mouthed vague characterisations of the blind (they 'see things in a more abstract manner than we do'), whereas Pignier opened out the pedagogy and allowed the students to breathe. At the New England Asylum for the Blind, Howe had heard of Haüy's efforts in Paris and visited Europe to investigate how institutions for the blind were organised. Pignier would constantly petition the government to increase the healthiness of the meals and the quality of the sleeping quarters for the students, and on his visit to the Institute, Howe registered his astonishment at the exposure of the students to independent outdoor activities:

> I have often observed with a delighted eye the movement of the blind boys in Paris as they leave the Institution to go to play; each grasps a cord held by a seeing boy, and follows him rapidly and unhesitatingly through narrow streets, until they enter the immense 'Garden of Plants' [*Jardin des Plantes*], when quitting the string they run among the trees, and frolic and play together with all the zest and enjoyment of seeing children. They know every tree and shrub, they careen it up one alley and down another, they chase, catch, overthrow and knock each other about, exactly like seeing boys; and to judge by their laughing faces, their wild and unrestrained gestures, and their loud and hearty shouts, they partake equally [in] the delightful excitement of boyish play. (Howe, in Mellor 2006: 60)

Pignier received Barbier and became convinced that his *écriture nocturne* would be of great value to the Institute. Although Barbier's system of punched coded messages was originally conceived for military use, his deep interest in exotic languages inspired him to further develop the system. To that end, in 1824 he had submitted a paper to the French Academy of Sciences entitled *Essai du noctographie chinoise et persane*

['An essay on Chinese and Persian noctography']. In 1830, his *Essai sur les aveugles* further detailed how his *écriture nocturne* could be adapted specifically for use by the blind. With the development of the system, and with Pignier as the new director, Barbier was received once again by the Institute in that same year.

In the 1820s the French army used Barbier's system for night-time battlefield communications. Small holes were punched in cardboard as a means of reading communications in the dark without having to use a light, thus avoiding the possibility of being spotted. Unlike previous relief printing systems based on a recognisable alphabet, Barbier's system was entirely arbitrary, using six raised marks in various sequential spatial arrangements, differentiated from any conventional association with Roman letters or type. A key feature of the system therefore lay in its constitution as abstract tactile signs. The sequential dots were arranged into a code based on a twelve-dot unit or 'cell' of two rows of six horizontal dots (Merry 1937: 275). Each combination of dots within the cell arrangement was mapped to a particular letter or phonetic sound. However, in the form presented by Barbier, the cell arrangement mapped imprecisely on to the area any fingertip could cover in a single touch. The administration of the Institute initially rejected it for this reason. Barbier and the pupils at the Institute persisted in refining the system. Its potential was clearly envisioned by Pignier and pupil number 70, the blind student Louis Braille.

Louis Braille became blind at the age of three and entered the Institution in 1819, aged ten. Because of competing tactile writing systems, relatively few works were available for an inquisitive blind scholar. Those that were involved letters hand-carved on wooden planks, inscribed into cardboard, cast in lead to form abbreviated versions of books or other short works, or printed through specially adapted presses *in relievo*. Both the act of production and the process of reading through solid materials was cumbersome and slow. With a number of non-standardised systems of literacy, blind students were bound into an asymmetrical relationship of tutelage, not just being told *how* to read but also *what* to read. The sighted decided what illustrious and morally improving works to translate into tactile script. For example, in Victorian Britain, so-called Visiting Societies flourished from the mid-1850s that employed sighted helpers to read with the blind, as the pedagogical historian Oliphant explains: 'the sighted helper "shared" the experience of the blind person in reading pre-selected, edifying texts' (2008: 67), utilising the cumbersome Moon type, a bulky Roman-based system that only encouraged dependency on the sighted.

In 1824, aged fifteen, Braille adapted Barbier's twelve-dot system into a six-dot one of his own devising, deploying embossed dots in a variety of patterns to form a code with sixty-three possible combinations. Each combination had a typographical equivalent, representing a specific letter of the alphabet, a number, or a punctuation mark. In the English Braille System there are 189 contractions and short form words. Since Braille was developed by a Frenchman, certain accommodations were necessary for translation into English. The French language does not contain the letter 'W', so in order to bring it to English-speaking countries a 'W' had to be adapted. In 1826 Braille became a teacher at the Institution in Paris, but he failed to publish his system until 1829. Perhaps because few of the teachers at the Institution were themselves blind, they were reluctant to teach using this tactile system, but the blind students readily accepted it. It was not until two years after Braille's death, in 1854, that the school where he studied and later taught formally adopted his system. As it started out in the classrooms, and was at first disapproved of by the sighted teachers, Braille was used primarily as a means for blind persons to communicate with each other in a written language, and it remained so until more systematic adoption within schools for the blind.

Of course, it was Barbier's method that Braille would refine into the system that bears his name. When Pierre Armand Dufau became director of the Institution in 1840 he appraised other methods in tactile writing emerging from Edinburgh and Philadelphia, before officially adopting Braille's system. Elsewhere in France there were rivalries concerning the different systems, until the Paris conference of 1878 voted to promote Braille as a universal system. Some flavour of the disarray is portrayed by Oliphant: 'Britain experienced "The Battle of the Types" while North America had its own "War of the Dots", as rival systems were promoted by their inventors' (2008: 72). For example, while the Missouri School for the Blind adopted Braille in 1860, it was not adopted universally across the United States until 1917, in a form that involved standardised contractions known as Grade II Braille, when the systems were eventually harmonised between the United Kingdom and the United States. Along the way the Braille system was modified and adapted by American institutions purportedly for greater efficiency, leading to such alternatives as New York Point, which transposed the Braille array on to its side, and American Braille which was developed at the Perkins Institute in 1868.

In Britain, a tactile writing system was proposed by William Moon in 1847. This was a hybrid system of raised print based on simplified alphabetical symbols that became known as the Moon system, a halfway stage between visual verisimilitude of letters and arbitrary tactile symbols like Braille (Merry 1937: 276). Meanwhile, a London surgeon named Thomas Armitage, who had lost his sight late in life, was largely responsible for founding the British and Foreign Blind Association, forerunner of the Royal National Institute for the Blind. His aim was to establish a body of international prestige and influence. The blind had always enjoyed the support of the elite to a far greater extent than other disabled groups, and Queen Victoria became the Association's first patron and the Bishop of London its president, while the vice-presidents included two dukes and three earls. Reporting on the initial meeting of its London-based counterpart, the superintendent of the New York Institute for the Education of the Blind wrote that there was a collective decision to make 'the vexed question of the best tactile alphabet' its first object of study, since there was unanimous agreement that 'all forms of the [raised] Roman or "line" letter systems are failures' (Wait 1868: 27). The British and Foreign Blind Association's first annual report contained the judgements of a carefully chosen panel on the types of tactile writing they had considered. The Lucas, Moon, and Frere systems were 'useful but imperfect', and whereas Roman type was universally condemned, Braille was confirmed as the best choice for a common system. It was quicker to read, less bulky to print, could be written in a frame, and was the only one suited to adapting music notation.

Reading Braille today

The tortuous path to universal adoption and worldwide standardisation in the nineteenth century meets a rather anti-climactic situation in the twentieth and into the twenty-first. Braille is currently the system of choice for around 10 per cent of blind readers, according to a report by the US National Federation of the Blind in 2009. According to the same report, Braille use peaked in the United States at around 50 per cent in the 1950s (Rubin 2009). Following its slow start in France from 1854, competition with other systems, uneven adoption in the United Kingdom and the United States in 1860, and almost universal adoption worldwide, the decline of Braille has been steep in the second half of the twentieth century. During this period, accelerated by such factors as changes to US federal law in 1974 guaranteeing public education for students with disabilities of all kinds, philosophies of education have stressed integration rather than segregation of blind and deaf students. Increasingly, technologies such as screen readers, which convert onscreen text into audio, have not only made works of literature available through computers, but virtually the entirety of the material accessible and distributed through the internet. Such technologies not only ease entry into computer-mediated communication for those with sensory impairments, but arguably help erase difference or feelings of otherness. Emails, online forums or blogs need not identify the writer or reader as blind or vision-impaired, for example. Conversely, blind and vision-impaired populations, including academics, can reach sighted publics through these forms. The learning and use of Braille may be increasingly unpopular among certain demographics in part because it accentuates and marks out their difference. Nevertheless, the narrative of Braille's historical emergence from among competing tactile writing systems reveals much about the ongoing relationship between vision and touch, of fingers and eyes. As a system of raised dots it permits certain efficiencies in communication that are consistent with forms of substitution between the senses, but there is a particularity to Braille as a system which enhances the rapidity of literacy compared to previous systems of raised or embossed letters. So here we might ask, how does Braille operate as a tactile communication system, and how does it employ translations between sensory modalities? Is literacy through touch as efficient as, or even functionally equivalent to, literacy through visual means?

On average a sighted reader can read and process 300 words per minute. Reading via audio descriptions, such as audio books or a sighted reader employed to read to a blind person, achieves 125 words per minute on average. With the use of a 'compressor' which speeds up audio recordings of speech for the blind to 275 words per minute, or alternatively speeding up digital audio playback, audio reading can approach sighted reading in terms of speed. However, tactile reading is considerably slower, reaching on average 100 words per minute, a third of the sighted rate (Hollins 1989: 73–6). If the greatest disparity in reading speed lies between visual reading and tactile reading, the explanation is partly physiological and partly cognitive. The fingertips have the densest concentration of touch receptors within the hands (see Cattaneo and Vecchi 2011: 30) and are therefore comparable to the fovea centralis at the back of the eye. Consequently we might posit a physiological analogy between the high-definition optical resolution of the fovea, and the highly discriminatory tactile sensing of the hands and fingertips. However, this need not entail any functional equivalence between fovea and fingertip, eyes and hands. Tactile reading is performed by a sweep of the fingertips, either one or both index fingers, but no other haptic information is acquired in the process. This means, first, that the fingertips present a smaller area of contact with the text than the eye. Secondly, this form of reading through contact is necessarily sequential or successive, compared to more simultaneous information presented to the eye, since in visual reading there are ten or more points of information taken in simultaneously, and therefore some ability to read ahead, check comprehension, or perform error correction on the fly. The difference in reading rate is somewhat ameliorated by a series of recognised contractions of words outlined in Grade II Braille, such as 'tm' for 'tomorrow' or 'lr' for 'letter'. However, any increase in reading speed is marginal, especially because the contracted forms might 'read' similarly to other letters, and so proportionately increase margins for error.

In terms of brain activity, visual, audio, and tactile reading involve similar areas of the brain. Whether or not there is a physiological analogy between fovea and fingertip, then, the functional equivalence between vision and touch in terms of reading is in fact verifiable. For both tactile reading in Braille and visual reading the temporal lobe of the left hemisphere becomes active (Hollins 1989: 77), an area that includes the auditory cortex but, more significantly, is involved in language comprehension and naming. This is presumably applicable to other forms of tactile reading, such as the systems of embossed letters that preceded Braille. Psychological studies of blind reading by Loomis (1981) conclusively demonstrated that the superiority of Braille lies in the pattern of the dots, being simpler and less prone to error than letters. Through a series of experiments with different tactile writing systems, including raised dots in the shapes of letters comparable to the Moon system, it was shown that the number of dots needed to represent a Braille cell (3.2 on average) was significantly fewer than the number of dots needed to symbolise Roman alphanumeric characters (8.6 on average). Thus the Braille system is two and a half times more efficient as a communication system. Nevertheless, this experimental data opens up fascinating potential pathways for retinal prostheses, as we shall see in the following chapter on technologies of sensory substitution. The ability to stimulate the visual cortex, either through tactile arrays on the back or tongue, or through direct implants into the retina, not only builds upon the long thread throughout this book on sensory translations between hands and eyes, of sensory substitutions of touch for vision, but also begins to question what a sensory modality actually is.

Chapter 7

Seeing with the Tongue: Sight through Other Means

In early September 2013 I visited a laboratory at the University of Pittsburgh Medical Center, and by pre-arrangement met a research subject, an ex-policeman who had become blind a few years previously. He sat at a table, put on some dark glasses with a small protruding lens, placed a small flat plastic device in his mouth, and proceeded to reach out and touch a series of small brightly coloured objects, including cubes and spheres. A twenty-first century Molyneux man. The videofeed from his glasses was being output on a nearby monitor, and I could see what his glasses were pointed at. The shapes on the monitor were being converted into an array of electrical patterns on the surface of his tongue, and although he could not see the objects with his eyes, he was feeling their shapes and responding appropriately. Soon, it was my turn. It didn't take long to put the equipment on, and after some acclimatisation I could start to discern objects in vague locations based on tingling patterns. If I looked to the left, the patterns would drift to the right side of the tongue; if I moved closer, the objects would increase in size on the tongue surface. With more time, I have been told, my brain would adapt, the accuracy would increase, and tasks such as reading letters and numbers, or playing games, would be possible. All through patterns of stimuli on a 20 × 20 array of electrodes on the tongue. This technology, which can make blind subjects 'see', is called the BrainPort™ V100 sensory substitution device.

Previously, the notion of 'seeing with the hands' was an analogy, a means by which Descartes could explain the mechanisms of sight. Likewise, the analogy of 'reading with the fingers' was applied to decoding tactile signs or mechanically augmented learning materials, such as Braille or tactile maps, through the fingertips. While the language of equivalence in those cases is largely a rhetorical flourish, this chapter's examination of technologies of sensory substitution will subject the suitability of such analogies to more scrutiny. Over the past few years there has been coverage in mainstream media, and discussion in the philosophy and psychology literature, of technologies that allow blind subjects to 'see' through the skin and the tongue. The key goal of sensory substitution systems is that, in the absence of one modality, another may be repurposed to provide equivalent information. We therefore revisit the Molyneux question insofar as it pertains to the underlying mechanism behind sensory substitution, to summon evidence from experimental studies with sensory substitution technologies, and therefore to question the relationship between sense modalities, especially the privileged association between touch and vision. Do certain sensory substitutions, whether aided by technology or not, indicate a more general theory of the senses (see Chirimuuta and Paterson 2014 for a more philosophically developed version of this 'meta-Molyneux question')? If Molyneux was specifically questioning Locke about the relationship between touch and vision, can this be generalised in any way to other modalities? Can the tasks of hearing, touching, and seeing be performed through other means, translated between different modalities, say?

First, some terminology and acronyms. There are various technologies of sensory substitution that engage the modalities of vision, audition, and tactility, depending on the missing or impaired sense. Generically these are termed 'sensory substitution systems' (SSS) (Lenay et al. 2003; Noë 2009), or 'sensory substitution devices' (SSD) (Deroy and Auvray 2014). This chapter concentrates principally on one system, the tactile-visual sensory substitution (TVSS) system, also known as the BrainPort™ (see Figures 7.1 and 7.2), and explores its functionality and some implications for the blind and severely vision-impaired. Direct stimulation of the auditory nerves was accomplished in the 1960s, and cochlear implants (also known as 'bionic ears') were approved in 1984 and provided to hundreds of thousands of deaf subjects. More recently, trials with retinal prostheses (known as 'bionic eyes') have been ongoing, with teams around the world using competing solutions for those with vision loss due to degenerating photoreceptors, as occurs in the disease retinitis pigmentosa (RP). Fundamentally, sensory substitution technologies transform stimuli characteristic of one sensory modality (for example, vision) into stimuli of another sensory modality (for example, touch). The system achieves this by means of an electronic sensor that converts ambient energy or information such as light or sound through an electronic coupling system that coordinates the activation of a stimulator array (Lenay et al. 2003: 276). From abstruse and innovative experiments in the 1960s by neuroscientist Paul Bach-y-Rita at the University of Madison-Wisconsin, who initially used unwieldy mechanical installations that fed optical information from a camera to a series of metal pins that imprinted patterns on the skin of the back, to more portable wearable electronic devices such as his later BrainPort™, which produces vibrotactile stimulation to the tongue, such technologies are active ongoing perceptual experiments rather than a restorative shortcut.

As the blind and vision-impaired know all too well, history is peppered with technologies offered either as aids or as potential 'solutions' to blindness, packages that promise much but deliver little, such as white canes with embedded GPS systems, examples of so-called Electronic Travel Aids (ETA), and bespoke magnifiers and reading machines. TVSS, however, offers a more integrated approach, and has the potential to reveal a great deal about ordinary processes of perception, as well as aspects of brain function including cortical plasticity, the ability of parts of the brain to be repurposed, temporarily or permanently, in order to fulfil other types of functionality. In other words, there is something genuinely novel about such sensory substitution devices, with the potential for investigating the underlying mechanisms of cross-modal transfer, and to problematise what 'seeing' without eyes consists in, and what a 'sense modality' is. If vision can be accomplished through other, technological means, what does this say about sight and the function of the eyes?

Rather than giving a straightforward overview of sensory substitution technologies, after discussing a few case studies we will evaluate how these technologies are advancing psychological and philosophical debates, fostering fresh questions about blindness and visual processes. The significance of TVSS has been revisited in philosophy and popular neuroscience recently, for example by Alva Noë in his *Action in Perception* (2004) and *Out of Our Heads* (2009), and Norman Doidge in *The Brain that Changes Itself* (2007), among others, using instances of sensory substitution technologies as empirical examples to test out theories of neurological plasticity. Although it is tempting to employ the term 'sensory substitution' for more routine transfer between modalities, or even for analogous use such as 'seeing with the hands', in fact it has a rather specific application. In neuroscientific literature, Lenay et al. explain that sensory substitution 'denotes the ability of the central nervous system to integrate devices of this sort, and to constitute through learning a new "mode" of perception' (2003: 276). Integrating technological devices into perceptual schemas in this way augments existing modalities and, irrespective of claims about neurological plasticity, the aim and promise of such technologies is to produce a functional equivalence between the senses. This is a claim highlighted tentatively in previous chapters, but which will be examined here in more detail.

On senses and modalities: updating Molyneux

Since the Molyneux question was first posed, we have been tracing how experiments, surgery, and other empirical findings have disproved or amended philosophical hypotheses about blindness and perception. Subsequent philosophical discussion between Locke and Berkeley, and by later figures such as Reid, pivoted on the possibility of a level of sensory abstraction before perceptions of objects become modality-specific. One of Berkeley's stated tasks in *An Essay Towards a New Theory of Vision* was 'to consider the difference there is betwixt the ideas of sight and touch, and whether there be any idea common to both senses' (*Vision* §1). The philosopher Gareth Evans (1985) presents his summary and solution of the Molyneux problem as a lesson in dealing with the senses in more fine-grained bodily terms, considering the integration of vision with other bodily perceptions and sensations including audition and kinaesthesia. Evans dismissed psychological interpretations of the problem through Lotze (1885) and latterly von Senden (1960), which denied that the blind have any concept of space whatsoever, since it is better to 'suppose that spatial concepts can be learned through the subject's capacity to *perceive* spatially' (1985: 377). Even without sight there is, for the blind subject, the possibility of the formation of 'simultaneous perceptual representations of his [sic] vicinity' (Evans 1985: 382), whether this occurs through acoustics, touch, or any combination of bodily movement and sensation. Senses other than sight are involved in providing the blind subject's sense of space and aid in navigation through that space.

With the ability to empirically test theories of cross-modal transfer and models of sensory substitution after Molyneux, there arises an opportunity to question the very notion of what a 'sense modality' actually is. If Molyneux asks specifically about transfer between the modalities of vision and touch for the blind, are there other pathways between modalities that provide comparable functionality for sensory impairments other than blindness, say? Or does this suggest a more general theory of perception after Molyneux? In other words, is the relationship between vision and touch neurologically privileged, or are pathways between each of the sense modalities equally exploitable and plastic? Are sensory substitutions between audition and vision, say an auditory-visual sensory substitution (AVSS) system, neurologically comparable or in some way equivalent to a tactile-visual (TVSS) system? Moreover, does this notion of cross-modal transfer assume the Aristotelian model of the five senses as distinct modalities, such that touch, vision, hearing, smell, and taste are coherent and distinct modalities in themselves, or are the senses interleaved, interconnected in more complex ways, folded into sensory subsystems in a way that might problematise the notion of a discrete modality as such?

Previous philosophical accounts of the senses have assumed that the presence in perception of an external spatial field is a component of our usual bodily awareness, and is a stable characteristic of sensory modalities. If the spatial field is associated especially with vision, the background awareness of our embodiment is associated more with touch (Martin 1992; O'Shaughnessy 1989). From this, Michael Martin (1992) argues against the possibility of a general theory of perception. However, recent findings about the plasticity of neural systems underlying sensory performance, including those using sensory substitution systems, challenge this assumption. Upon experiencing optically driven touch stimulation in TVSS systems – the conversion of visual information into patterns of vibrotactile input on the skin – subjects develop a more corporeal or haptic awareness attuned to spatial navigation and orientation tasks. This would initially suggest that sensory systems are reconfigurable, and therefore that the Molyneux question about vision and touch could be extended to other senses. In other words, this opens up the possibility of cross-modal transfer of information between any sense modality, as evidenced by the fact that blind subjects are able to achieve complex spatial tasks through augmented video feeds and vibrotactile feedback. Yet, although there is extensive plasticity of sensory pathways, we cannot simply assume endless reconfigurability, and the inherent similarity of certain visual and haptic spatial functions makes these more 'substitutable' than other modalities. Experimental evidence will later show that touch and vision have a privileged relation, which should be unsurprising given the pervasive historical analogues and associations throughout this book.

If certain channels between modalities are privileged, especially between vision and touch, we must ask to what extent other modalities can be involved in substitutions without making invalid generalisation. One factor which motivates this question is the growing appreciation of the importance of cross-modal spatial attention (see Spence and Driver 2004) and cross-modal sensations that cannot be understood within modality-specific theories, such as bodily sensations that lie outside the Aristotelian model of the five distinct or extant senses (e.g. Kemp and Fletcher 1993; Spelke 1998; Streri and Gentaz 2004; Ganson and Ganson 2010). Moreover, this work is clearly complementary to the ongoing debate over how the sense modalities should be categorised and defined (e.g. Keeley 2002; 2009; Noë 2004). Much empirical work suggests that each modality is more complex and disunified than our everyday embodied experience suggests. So we should remain open to the possibilities afforded by a theoretical reintegration of the senses. Even though the idea of sensory substitution is promising, especially as investigated through emerging technologies, we already know that the modalities are not ultimately unified or fully substitutable. There are also significant findings of disunity within modalities. Given this, we observe that some functionally defined components (i.e. sub-modalities) do share commonalities with other modalities. These commonalities can be enhanced with perceptual learning, the BrainPort™ being an excellent example of sensory accommodation and learning that allows for sense substitution. Through examining such technologies we can discern something of the boundaries and alliances involved between the senses, and delineate effective examples of 'functional equivalences' between the senses. If the BrainPort™ encourages us to 'see' through the skin or the tongue, what kind of 'seeing' is this, exactly?

Sensory substitutions

Each of the sense modalities achieves a number of tasks, and some are common to other modalities. If perspective, distance, and the movement of an object towards us is seen through the eyes, for example, these are not simply patterns of light on the retina but are cognitively processed as perspective or movement, as opposed to shadows, colours, and lines cast on to a photoreceptive layer of the eye. In the absence of light, those interpretations of the properties of objects are achieved through other, non-visual, means. As we will see, the mechanism of sensory substitution relies on co-opting certain processing streams in the substituting sense, the ones most similar to the substituted sense, due to functional similarities or correspondences within subsystems.

Following Berkeley to a large extent, and consciously echoing the differentiation between a cube and a sphere that the Molyneux subject must determine, one of Martin's (1992) main points was that the geometric curvature of a rubber ball is *seen* in the context of a visual field, but *felt* as a type of impression on the skin, an impingement upon the bodily contour. His assumption is that these contrasting characteristics of the modalities, what is seen and what is felt, are fixed. But here is where technologies of sensory substitution can advance the debate. What if, under certain circumstances, the experience of touch can be released from its entanglement with bodily sensation, to become more distal and vision-like? In other words, does the changeability of sensory systems, and the variety of perceptions they bring about, mean there is no neat or fixed separation between visual and tactile spatial perception?

Of course, there has been a range of both empirical and theoretical work that challenges the fixity of the modalities. It would be disingenuous to portray the positions of figures like Révész and Martin as representative of any academic discipline, for within a similar time period there has already been phenomenologically influenced work on haptics that contests these views (for further discussion see Paterson 2007). In an oft-cited paper on active touch, for example, the ecological psychologist James J. Gibson (1962) describes the key role of purposeful movement, when the sense of touch is used for gathering information about the shape of objects. When subjects were engaged in such 'active touch' tasks they were unable to report the flux of sensations on the skin, only the rigid edges of the object felt. He states: 'One perceives the object-form but not the skin-form. The latter is, in fact, continually changing as the fingers move in various ways. It is almost completely unreportable, whereas the pattern of physical corners and edges seems to emerge in experience' (1962: 482). In active touch, *contra* Martin, there is no body-field as such, and the perception lands firmly on the external object being perceived. For example, when changing gear in a car with manual transmission, we direct our attention less to the surface texture of the gearstick, and more to the pattern of muscular movement necessary to achieve the requisite gear change. Gibson contrasts reports of active touch with his subjects' observations of passive touch, cases where the experimenter induces the same tactile sensations as would be caused by the subject's manual exploration. In those cases the cutaneous events become distinct to the subject as something happening to the body surface. Gibson concludes that there is a mode of touching that is vision-like. Seemingly in direct answer to those like Révész and Martin who assume the separation and fixity of the modalities, Gibson observes:

> vision and touch have nothing in common *only when they are conceived as channels for pure and meaningless sensory data*. When they are conceived instead as channels for information-pickup, having active and exploratory sense organs, they have much in common. (1962: 490; original emphasis)

This line of thought will be explored in the following section. What Gibson acknowledges is the possibility of an inherent flexibility in the way that sensory modalities represent external objects and bodily occurrences. This flexibility is what is exploited in technologies of sensory substitution.

The case of the 'seeing' tongue

Sensory substitution technologies require fast perceptual learning and, over the long term, substantial cortical re-mapping. There is a range of such sensory substitution systems, including tactile-audio and tactile-vestibular substitution, but the system most relevant to the Molyneux question is tactile-visual sensory substitution (TVSS), as it foregrounds the translation between vision and touch, especially when performing spatial tasks. The pioneer of TVSS from the 1960s until his death in 2006 was the neuroscientist Paul Bach-y-Rita who, in a landmark book *Brain Mechanisms in Sensory Substitution*, neatly summarises the aims of a TVSS system: 'In a tactile sensory substitution approach, a sensory system previously virtually restricted to contact information must mediate three-dimensional spatial information and integrate spatial cues originating at a distance' (1972: 66).

The first devices in Bach-y-Rita's laboratory were largely mechanical, such as the hulking research device built in 1968 that translated a tripod-based low-resolution video feed into patterns of pressure on the skin. Because of the physical size of the tactile array, a 20 × 20 grid of solenoid stimulators was originally built into a dentist's chair with a heavy base, and the research subject manipulated a large, zoomable television camera on a tripod in order to scan objects on a table in front (Bach-y-Rita et al. 1969: 963). Training with blind research subjects concentrated initially on solid geometrical shapes and easily discernible lines, and even in this primitive incarnation, given sufficient numbers of hours in training, there was the potential to understand the visual rules of perspective and occlusion, for 'learning to see':

> With repeated presentations [of objects through the device], the latency or time-to-recognition of these objects falls markedly; in the process, the students discover visual concepts such as perspective, shadows, shape distortion as a function of viewpoint, and apparent change in size as a function of distance. (Bach-y-Rita et al. 1969: 963)

The next version implanted the 20 × 20 array on to the trunk of the body, the only practicable area due to the 10-inch size of the array, for more portability (Bach-y-Rita 1972: 3). Despite such low resolution, with periods of training congenitally blind subjects could actually discern basic shapes and letters. The transition to progressively more portable solutions necessitated a shift from mechanical to electrical systems, and in 1971 a prototype of the so-called Smith-Kettlewell Portable Electrical Stimulation System was demonstrated, with blind subjects using a head-mounted camera, but with a lower resolution 8 × 8 array of brass discs held in a plastic grid pressed to the abdomen. An unforeseen outcome of this increased mobility was the potential for the subject to interact with the environment, so that picking up a telephone, for example, exploited a 'hand-sensor' coordination that was technically impossible before. Succeeding versions of these devices unsurprisingly decreased in physical size while increasing the resolution of the vibrotactile array and were subsequently developed for commercial use, marketed in the early 1990s as the VideoTact™ for $45,000 (Visell 2009).

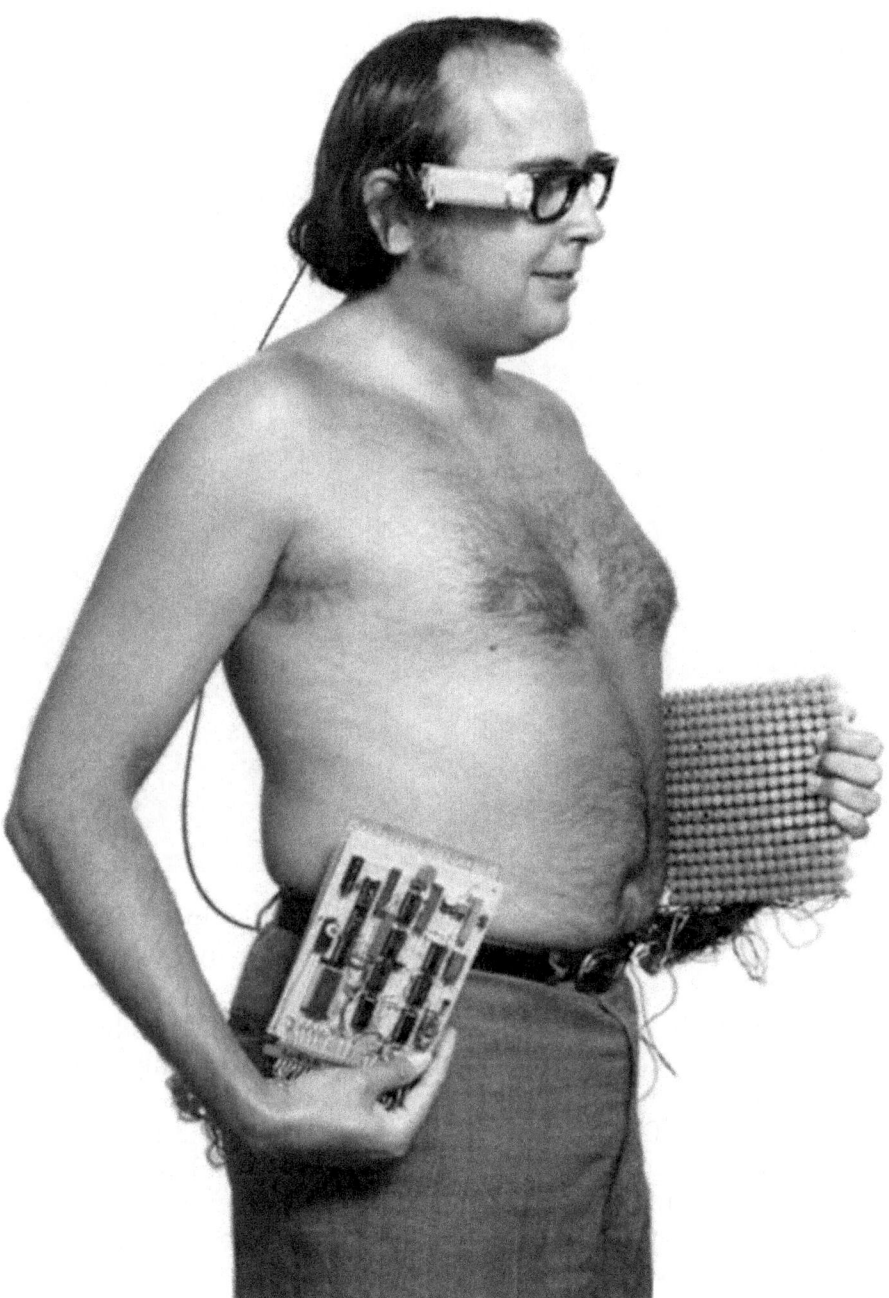

Figure 7.1 An early incarnation of Bach-y-Rita's TVSS system, with a tactile array for the abdomen.

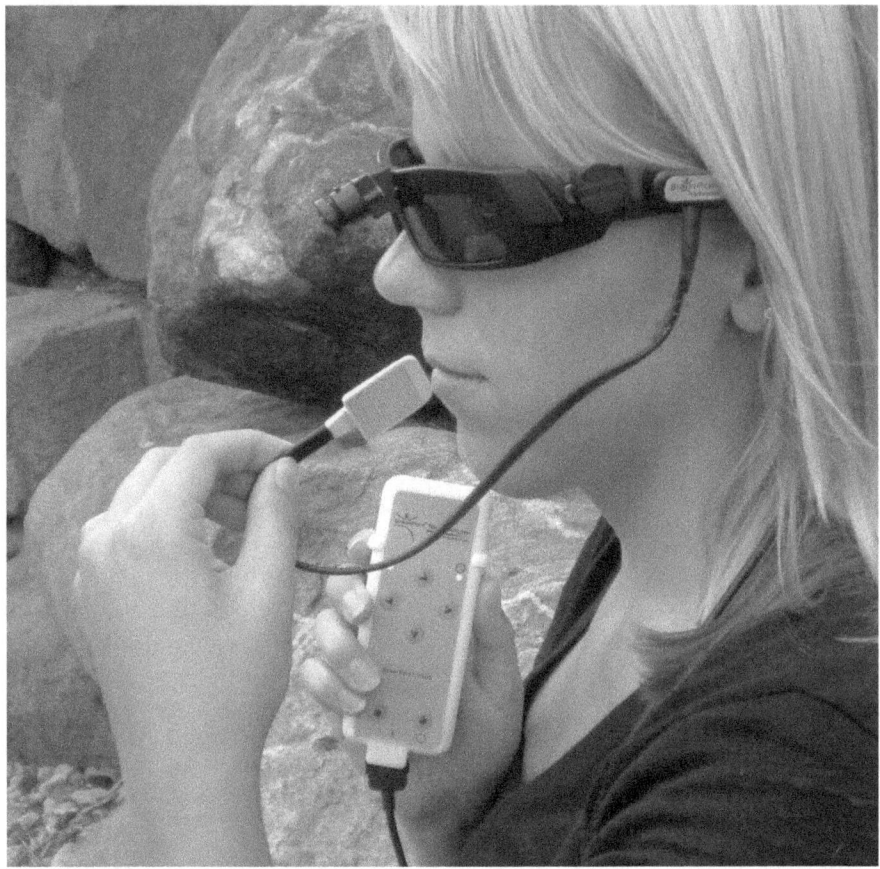

Figure 7.2. The BrainPort™ V100 so-called 'lollipop' TDU developed by Bach-y-Rita through his company Wicab.

More recently a tongue-based variant known colloquially as the 'lollipop' has been tested experimentally. Developed initially by Bach-y-Rita and his company Wicab Inc. from 1998, the lollipop is a highly portable Tongue Display Unit (TDU), marketed as the BrainPort™ V100. The trademark and the use of the term 'BrainPort' might be thought significant, heralding the promise of a series of technologies that bypass sensory limitations. A quote from Wicab's online promotional video encourages this interpretation, claiming that 'your brain is what really sees, not your eyes' (Wicab.com 2011), an almost exact paraphrase of the Cartesian sentiment from *Dioptrique*, 'it is the mind which sees, not the eye; and it can see immediately only through the intervention of the brain' (Descartes 1965: 108). The idea is that the TVSS technology creates a new portal into the brain, allowing it to 'see' again. It implies that the senses are interchangeable in that touch mechanisms can be transformed into visual ones. It is simply a case of directing optical information to the skin, from where it will be channelled to the brain. Because of neural plasticity, the brain can use information from the tongue as if it came from the eye.

The BrainPort™ has had some coverage in news media, memorably through a profile of a British soldier, Craig Lundberg, who was blinded in a rocket-propelled grenade attack in Iraq in 2007. In 2010 Lundberg was involved with trials of the technology, and this raised the profile of the TDU or 'lollipop' in the British media, including TV news and newspaper stories. 'He was told he would never "see" again. But now he can – with his tongue' was one by-line in the *Huffington Post* (Smith 2010). And, in a way that complements Bach-y-Rita's summary of how three-dimensional cues are interpreted from two-dimensional cutaneous sensations, an article in *The Guardian* about Lundberg explains this to a non-specialist readership: 'The BrainPort converts visual images into a series of electrical pulses which are sent to the tongue, the different strength of the tingles can be read or interpreted so the user can mentally visualise their surroundings and navigate around objects' (Bowcott 2010: 13).

Sensory substitution devices like the 'lollipop' clearly have the potential for rehabilitation from ophthalmic injuries and acquired blindness for the public as well as the military. This is not like Braille, and this is not seeing with the skin of the fingertips. Instead, a small videocamera mounted in the frames of dark spectacles streams video footage into a small belt-mounted computer that converts the signal into a flexible 25×25 electrode array. Like a small retainer it can be freely inserted or removed from the mouth. When placed directly upon the tongue, patterns of electrical stimulation through the array feel like champagne bubbles popping with different intensities in different places, changing according to updates in the videostream. This system outperforms earlier versions of TVSS because the tongue is smaller and more sensitive than the back or abdomen, and saliva in the mouth enhances the electrolytic environment, increasing conductivity (Bach-y-Rita et al. 1998). The technology has proved successful for seeing shapes, letters, reading words, and enhancing mobility and spatial awareness without vision. Footage of blind subjects playing games of noughts and crosses, throwing darts at dartboards, and navigating cluttered courses featured in the TV news and on the BrainPort™ website, and confirms what earlier trials in the laboratory had found, that the specifications of resolution and refresh rate for the tactile array are 'good enough' to make the device useful in practical tasks (Sampaio et al. 2001; Ptito et al. 2005).

The technology has already attracted much philosophical interest. Heil (1983), Hurley and Noë (2003), and Noë (2004) all describe TVSS as endowing a kind of seeing. In fact, blindness and the TVSS feature in Noë's *Action in Perception* (2004) in order to bolster his overall thesis of an enactive theory of perception. Nevertheless, along the way he also supports the position taken here and by Millar, that 'we cannot individuate perceptual modalities by physical or physiological criteria alone', and that TVSS demonstrates exactly this because 'TVSS is a mode of quasi-seeing without any involvement of eyes or visual cortex' (2006: 111). Morgan (1977) wrote a largely historical overview of the Molyneux question, but in his final chapter on technologies for the blind he included an account of an early incarnation of Bach-y-Rita's TVSS experiments. A positive answer to the question was implied, that touching through a TVSS was comparable in significant ways to seeing. One of the reasons for claiming that TVSS enables a kind of seeing is the functional equivalences between different modalities, effectively illustrated in the 'looming' effect of a camera zoom. Bach-y-Rita himself had noticed during trials that if the experimenter makes the TVSS camera zoom into an object, the sudden felt expansion of the object through stimulation on the tongue causes subjects to flinch, just as if the object were hurtling towards them (1972: 98). This zoom-like effect relies on a characteristically visual stimulus, what Gibson (1979) terms the expansion of optic flow. In this case TVSS enables the modality of touch to respond to spatial cues normally only available to vision, but whether these particular functional equivalences should rightly be described as 'seeing' or 'sight' is debatable.

Another reason these TVSS systems are unlike Braille is that the subject need not be blind or even vision-impaired for there to be vision-like perceptions through the tongue, or for the zooming effect to work. As noted based on my own experience, for both blind and sighted it takes a period of acclimatisation to the machinery. Switching on the machinery does not immediately endow the subject with any new perceptual capacity. Instead, there is a steady learning process through which the TVSS system becomes a useful means of performing certain perceptual operations (Bach-y-Rita 1972; Sampaio et al. 2001; Ptito et al. 2005; Bubic et al. 2010). The learning rates for different tasks vary. While target detection and spatial orientation are almost immediate, discrimination of horizontal and vertical lines and direction of movement takes some practice. The fast recognition of ordinary objects usually takes ten hours of learning, according to Lenay et al. (2003: 279). A crucial pre-condition for learning to take place is that the subject must be allowed to manipulate the camera and actively engage with the sequence of image capturing. A series of static forms on the tactile matrix does not facilitate learning, and feedback on discriminatory performance is essential (Sampaio 1995). This chimes in with Gibson's (1979) observations on 'active' and 'passive' touch, above. Following this process of adaptation, and consistent with Gibson's distinction between feeling an object as opposed to feeling its disparate outlines and contours, the tactile stimulation which conveys information about distal objects is readily distinguished from local irritations on the skin due to the electrode matrix. Furthermore, TVSS stimulation is not felt as if 'on' the skin, as a kind of bodily sensation, but comes to be 'projected' into a reference frame or field external to the immediate point of vibrotactile contact with the device. What might seem surprising is that this effect does not require a particularly sophisticated system or a dense tactile array, and was notable even in the earliest incarnation of Bach-y-Rita's TVSS in the dentist's chair:

> Our subjects spontaneously report the external localization of stimuli, in that sensory information seems to come from in front of the camera, rather than from the vibrotactors on their back. Thus, after sufficient experience, the use of the vision substitution system seems to become an extension of the sensory apparatus. (Bach-y-Rita et al. 1969: 964)

In other words, through acclimatisation with the equipment, the tactile-cutaneous field comes to be interpreted as a visuo-spatial field.

Lenay et al (2003: 282) describe an even more pared-down system used in their laboratory, with a single photodiode on the index finger of one hand, and a vibrator on the index finger of the other. Once the subject experiences the correlations between exploratory movement, object presence, and tactile stimulation, the vibrations induce perception of a distal object even with this single point of contact. Furthermore, Lenay's team note that the position of the vibrator on the hand can be altered without affecting the perceived location of the distal object. As they write, 'Initially, the subject only feels a succession of stimulations on the skin. But after the learning process [...] the subject ends up neglecting these tactile sensations, and is aware only of stable objects at a distance, "out there" in front of him [sic]' (Lenay et al. 2003: 279). TVSS users perceive objects as residing in a space removed from immediate contact which, in this regard, is analogous to the visual field. This observation evidently contrasts with Martin's hypothesis above that objects felt by touch must appear as impingements on the bodily contour, but not contained within the sense field of that modality. As Lenay et al. continue,

> the subject appears to ignore the position of the tactile stimulations [...] to the benefit of an apprehension of the spatial position of the light source. Conversely, artificial stimuli produced independently of the movement of the finger on which the photoelectric cell is placed are not associated with a distal perception, but continue to be perceived proximally at the level of the skin. Similarly, if the movements [of the perceiver] cease, the distal spatial perception disappears. (2003: 282)

That the effect requires only a TVSS of the most minimal sort is notable, as it shows that spatial perception of objects within a field comparable to a visual field can arise with sensory capacities that otherwise bear little resemblance to vision. In addition, the simplicity of the equipment underlines the starkness of the translation from cutaneous stimulation into a visuo-spatial field with distance, and underlines once again the significance of Gibson's 'active' touch within exploratory movement. Once the subject experiences the correlations between exploratory movement, object presence, and tactile stimulation, the vibrations induce the perception of a distal object, even when the position of the vibrator on the hand is altered.

What happens during the periods of acclimatisation with the sensory substitution equipment? More precisely, what is happening to the brain during this learning process? The learning required for TVSS use is understood to be correlated with structural and physiological changes in the brain, including the visual cortex. In one neuroimaging study, Ptito, Moesgaard, and Gjedde (2005) trained eleven early blind subjects to locate an object using the 12 × 12 electrode 'lollipop' or tongue display unit (TDU). After one hour of practice the blind participants showed significantly increased activity in the visual cortex when performing the task, activity not found in the PET scans prior to training. In other words, learning to use TVSS involved the recruitment of new sensory areas of the brain that were not activated initially. It is interesting to compare this study with the longstanding observation that Braille reading involves the recruitment of the visual cortex, even in blindfolded sighted participants undergoing prolonged visual deprivation (Kauffman et al. 2002; Pascual-Leone et al. 2006).

Neuroplasticity in sensory substitution

The findings about the re-ordering of cortical activity are unsurprising. As Bach-y-Rita and Kercel declare: 'Sensory substitution is [...] only possible because of brain plasticity' (2003: 541). The fact that the brain is 'plastic' throughout its lifespan, rather than fixed after a critical period as Weisel and Hubel had assumed, is increasingly recognised to be key to understanding many of its functions, not only in memory and learning, but also for perceptual and cognitive processes, and of course recovery after injury. Bach-y-Rita was one of the earliest proponents of this now fashionable idea, based on his observations in neuro-rehabilitative medicine, sparked by an incapacitating stroke that his father experienced but eventually recovered from (Doidge 2007: 20). Profound changes in the organisation of sensory systems occur not only after contact with substitution devices, but also as a result of sensory loss or temporary sensory deprivation (Büchel et al. 1998; Kauffman et al. 2002; Pascual-Leone et al. 2006; Merabet and Pascual-Leone 2010; Bubic et al. 2010). It is now scientifically accepted that the brains of non-sighted individuals compensate by recruiting visual areas in tactile and auditory tasks, and the extent of compensation does indeed correlate with enhanced behavioural performance.

Certain blind individuals, most famously Daniel Kish, have learned to navigate through unfamiliar spaces using an echolocation technique, emitting clicking noises with the tongue and attending to the echoes in order to sense approaching obstacles. This skill develops over time and can be learned, and indeed Kish runs training workshops to teach echolocation to blind subjects. Kish himself makes the distinction between the modalities and their proximal and distal qualities that we have encountered with TVSS, in this case prioritising audition and the spatial properties of acoustics. In an ABC News article tellingly entitled 'Like a bat, blind man uses sound to "see"', Kish explains in his own words: 'We can kind of think of echolocation as being sort of far vision; it's good for things that are far away and off the ground [...] The cane is good for things that are nearer and at ground level' (in Moisse 2011). This repurposing of parts of the visual cortex for other tasks has been verified in the laboratory. Thaler, Arnott, and Goodale (2011) have published fMRI data on Kish, who lost his sight in childhood, and another subject who lost their sight in adolescence, indicating that the primary visual cortex is involved in the utilisation of echo information for detecting objects in space. In other words, the self-motivated learning of echolocation has caused the visual cortex to become involved in a non-visual spatial task, just like a TVSS system. Neuroplasticity can involve changes in the number and strength of synaptic connections, metabolic changes, and even the growth of new neurons (*neurogenesis*) in the adult brain, although neurogenesis is not implicated in sensory substitution. What is essential for the effective operation of TVSS is either the growth or reinforcement of peripheral connections from the substituting modality (touch or audition, in the above cases) to the central brain areas which typically receive information from vision. This allows for the substituting modality to receive stimulation in a format that is unusual for that modality – for example, the optic flow information in TVSS, above – and for that stimulus to be interpreted in an appropriate way, in this case, as a 'looming' object.

Other experiments involving the surgical rewiring of sensory pathways to the cortex demonstrate the brain's ability to alter in response to changes in perceptual input. Mriganka Sur and his team at Massachusetts Institute of Technology operated on newborn ferrets in one brain hemisphere, re-routing the optic nerve previously connected to the visual cortex to the auditory cortex, the brain area associated with audition (Noë 2009: 53–4). Some might assume that, upon waking, the ferrets would hear with their eyes, but of course Sur's team showed instead that they experienced vision through the auditory cortex. The link between brain areas, in this case the visual and auditory cortices, and their associated sensory experiences, was demonstrated to be plastic or malleable. Not only is this an impressive illustration of cortical plasticity but, through the observation of the ferrets seeing with the auditory cortex, it suggests an underlying functional equivalency. As Bavelier and Neville write: 'Such results confirm that sensory inputs have a central role in specifying the functional architecture of the brain regions that they contact' (2002: 445). In other words, as in the neonatal ferrets, the brain will reorganise its usual functional areas in order to accommodate a deprivation of sensory input, such as blindness or deafness. But this neuroplasticity is not limited to neonates. Significant levels of plasticity have been observed in experiments involving mature animals, although not on the same scale as the neonatal mammals (Rauschecker and Kniepert 1994; van Brussel et al. 2011). Nevertheless, it is still true to say that the immature brain has a degree of plasticity that is lost to the adult one. Accordingly Bubic et al. (2010: 368) recommend introduction to sensory substitution devices as early as possible in childhood to maximise the potential benefit.

Sensory substitution is possible because of functional similarities across certain modalities, and can be thought of as expanding the repertoire of tasks for which touch uses object-centred representations. But not all functions within modalities are comparable, and this highlights the inevitable limitations of physiological factors when comparing not just eyes with hands, but also eye movements with hand movements. This is because plasticity also occurs in motor areas of the brain, regions involved in orchestrating the movements of eyes and hands. As we have seen, acclimatisation and practice in controlling the TVSS camera is crucial to developing proficiency. This is because perception is at least in part a sensory-motor skill (Findlay and Gilchrist 2003; Noë 2004). So, to substitute seeing for touch, the subject must learn a pattern of movements that optimises the capture of visual information in TVSS, and these must become automatic through long-term structural changes in the brain. The blind subject's active control of the TVSS camera is a requirement for learning to interpret the vibrotactile patterns. Efficient manipulation of the camera is essential for strong perceptual performance, a sensorimotor skill that develops with prolonged use of TVSS. However, if the subject's viewpoint is controlled through directing the head-mounted camera, this involves always pointing the camera towards a scene in order to interpret it, and therefore continually orienting the head in its entirety. This will never be as fluid or rapid as the automatic and largely unconscious control of eye movements that we perform every day to fill in a visual scene in terms of central and peripheral vision. Saccades, the type of eye movement used for most visual tasks such as scanning scenes, examining objects, and reading, are actually the fastest movements made by the human body. An adult engaged in a natural viewing task makes 3–5 saccades each second, and saccadic reaction times can be as short as 100 milliseconds (Fischer and Weber 1993), whereas the minimum reaction time for a manual response is more than twice as long at 250 milliseconds (Kirchner and Thorpe 2006). The oculomotor system, which involves the unconscious muscular control of the eye's saccades, performs an extremely active perceptual process that TVSS systems are unlikely to replicate in the near future. If likened to a blind man's cane, this would be an exceptionally rapid, continual, and spatially variegated prodding of a cane in order to determine the contents of the scene, and to accommodate any changes or updates in that scene. The lesson here concerns the limits of sensory substitution, and the differentiated functionality of the sense organs and their associated sensorimotor subsystems. Until camera control can approach the precision and rapidity of sighted oculomotor control, TVSS enhanced touch will never be fully functionally equivalent to vision.

TVSS may never be exactly functionally equivalent to vision, but improvements in video resolution and the tactile array promise richer experiences of 'seeing' for the blind. These improvements can only go so far, however, as there is an enormous difference in the spatial resolution of pressure receptors on the skin compared with photoreceptors in the eye. So even if technological advances deliver TDUs with a far higher resolution than the current 25 × 25 available, the device will meet the inherent limits of human vibrotactile discrimination and the density of nerve endings in the associated body parts. Despite the possibilities of neurosensory structural reorganisation, the number and distribution of cutaneous nerve endings is physiologically fixed and not subject to plasticity. Bach-y-Rita and Kercel (2003) argue that such low tactile resolution is not actually an obstacle to TVSS replacing sight, but this is the case only if one constrains the definition of sight to certain coarse discriminations or optically induced responses, such as the recognition of large projected shapes against a dark background, or the ability to dodge a looming object. The acuities attained through earlier incarnations of the 'lollipop', as reported by Sampaio et al. (2001), remain relatively limited, as a sighted person performing at this level would be classified legally blind. Moreover recent media coverage showing impressive feats performed with TVSS (for example, the BBC's *Click*, 2010, and the *The Brain: A Secret History*, 2011) also reveal the intensity of concentration necessary to accomplish tasks that the sighted take for granted.

Despite the physiological limitations, the case studies and experimental findings contest the assumptions articulated earlier through Révész and Martin that the spatial properties of sensory systems are fixed and ultimately incommensurable. The point is that when the sense of touch is presented with information which was optical in origin, and trained to respond to these stimuli, new connections are forged between areas of the brain involved in touch and those normally involved in vision. A consequence is that the touch modality becomes more 'vision-like', especially in its representation of the spatial location of objects at a distance from the body. And, following Gibson, just as a visual image is not felt as a local irritation of the retina, a TVSS image is not felt as a stimulation of the skin. The sense of touch need not literally feel in touch with the objects it perceives. Against the previous assumptions of incommensurate sensory-spatial fields, then, through TVSS the sense usually characterised as proximal can indeed become distal. As such, the cross-modal plasticity observed following TVSS reveals something of the inherent complexity of the touch modality, in terms of how it represents objects in space, and again prompts us to question the limits of what a modality supposedly 'is', given the neuroplasticity we have seen, and the shifting relationship between the sense organs and their sensorymotor subsystems.

Lessons in sensory substitution from Braille

Having acknowledged that no general claims can be made about the individual senses because of their changeability, but that plasticity is observed in sensory systems following TVSS, we can see parallels from another low-tech form of tactile-visual sensory substitution, Braille. The ability to read Braille is shaped by certain functional commonalities between touch and vision which are robust, since we saw multiple systems of tactile scripts arise and compete with each other. This robustness indicates the relative stability of neurological architectures through which functional equivalences may occur, so where is the place for plasticity? This section surveys some of the neurological literature on Braille learning in order to answer the question. Along the way, we realise the surprising extent of activity in the visual cortex in reading Braille.

Conventional writing itself is a sensory substitution technology, efficiently converting aural phonemes into visual graphemes or pictograms. Braille, in turn, re-codes the visual alphabet into manually perceptible sequences of characters. Here it is significant that sighted people find it virtually impossible to learn to read Braille by touch. Those sighted subjects who do learn Braille end up relying on the visual rather than haptic recognition of the characters. Significantly, however, blind Braille readers employ areas of the visual cortex for this activity (Cohen et al. 1997; Hamilton and Pascual-Leone 1998). Further studies have shown that activity in the visual cortex is actually necessary and not merely incidental. Braille readers receiving transcranial magnetic stimulation (TMS) scans which disrupt activity in the visual cortex find that they are temporarily unable to distinguish the characters (Kupers et al. 2007). James et al. (2006) report that an extremely proficient Braille reader who suffered a stroke to the visual cortex lost her ability completely.

A series of papers involving haptics researchers Lederman and Klatzky (e.g. Lederman et al. 1990; Klatzky et al. 1985; Klatzky and Lederman 2003) show that it is surprisingly difficult to recognise a two-dimensional raised line drawing of an everyday object by touch alone, something we do effortlessly and instantaneously by sight. We touch to recognise shapes and objects in a different way than looking with the eyes: 'haptic object identification cannot rely virtually entirely on information about the spatial layout of edges, as appears to be the case in vision, because spatial information is extracted coarsely and slowly by means of touch' (Klatzky and Lederman 2003: 116). Put simply, the message is that the kind of information that is best for visual stimulation is not optimal for touch. In drawings, the two-dimensional projection of a three-dimensional object is decoded by the visual system easily, whereas the haptic system struggles to make sense of this kind of spatial representation.

Conversely, other kinds of spatial tasks are more easily achieved through touch, especially when plasticity allows for the recruitment of new brain areas to perform them. It turns out that in Braille, just as with TVSS, the learning process through which touch is involved in a new kind of spatial discrimination does involve plasticity, and this is a reorganisation within the visual cortex. Earlier we noted the difficulty for sighted subjects in learning Braille, but as Pascual-Leone and his team (2006) report, in certain circumstances they *can* learn to read Braille haptically, and visual cortical plasticity is observed, but only if they spend a week under conditions of complete visual deprivation, and are provided ample training in Braille use. Plasticity is therefore absolutely crucial in the sensory substitution involved in Braille, and occurs relatively rapidly in the blind or the blindfolded. However, for the blindfolded (sighted) subjects this cortical reorganisation disappears rapidly, typically within 24 hours of the blindfolds being removed.

There is one more remarkable thing from Pascual-Leone's research which has profound implications for blind and sighted subjects alike, and returns us to the earlier question about what constitutes a modality as opposed to a sense. Their results suggest that the tactile input to the visual cortex already exists in the sighted, but is ordinarily 'masked' by visual input and activity, since clearly there was insufficient time in the experiment for entirely new neural pathways to grow. The rapidity of the cortical reorganisation, in other words, highlights a set of preexisting coordinations between parts of the visual and somatosensory (tactile) cortices, so that submodalities of touch and of vision effect functional equivalences. As Pascual-Leone et al. summarise:

> [A] sense-specific brain region like the 'visual cortex' may be visual only because we have sight and because the kinds of computations performed by the striate cortex [AKA primary visual cortex, or 'V1'] are best suited for retinal, visual information. For example, we might

postulate that the 'visual cortex' is involved in discriminating precise spatial relations of local, detail[ed] features of an object or scene, which might be more advantageously done using visual than other sensory modalities. However, in the face of visual deprivation or well-chosen, challenging tasks, the striate cortex may unmask its tactile and auditory inputs to implement its computational functions on the available nonvisual sensory information. (2006: 173)

What emerges is the idea that certain perceptual functions can be characterised non-modally, whether tracking nearby objects through a TVSS or the precise spatial location of Braille dots on a page. Whether the 'input' for this task is provided by one sensory modality or another, the implication is that 'processing' need not be served by a modality-specific brain region. Ordinarily, some modalities are better suited to providing this input than others. So even if visual input dominates when the visual system is intact, the function need not be thought of as necessarily 'visual' per se, since in temporary or permanent blindness another modality can substitute for vision and perform the function. Earlier assumptions (e.g. by Révész and Martin) that each sense is monothematic or uniform in its representation of space are replaced with a more plastic model in which modalities contain within themselves numerous functional streams requiring different spatial reference frames, some of which may be translatable to those of other modalities.

To sum up the argument of the previous sections, the apparent interchangeability of senses is not due to an unconstrained plasticity, but rather the plastic reinforcement of one aspect of the substituting modality (e.g. fine spatial discrimination in an external spatial reference frame) that was pre-existent, but overshadowed by the substituted modality. Although the role of neuroplasticity was highlighted, Pascual-Leone has shown there may well be pre-existing cross-modal pathways which already have pre-established functional equivalences. Based on the investigation of TVSS systems it is clear that there is no irreconcilable difference between vision and touch, if within each of these modalities there are various functional streams, some of which do comparable things haptically as are typically done visually. One of the key common functional points of comparison between individual modalities lies in their representation of objects in space. There is variety and some interchangeability in the spatial reference frames employed by each individual modality. Touch, as well as vision, may equally use object-centred (allocentric) rather than body-centred (egocentric) frames of reference (Millar 2006; Klatzky 1998) for certain tasks. Sensory substitution is possible because of (possibly pre-existing) functional similarities across modalities, and in the case of TVSS involves expanding the repertoire of tasks for which touch uses object-centred representations, therefore providing a visuo-spatial 'scene' for the blind subject through touch, or indeed the tongue.

Conclusion: touch-like vision and vision-like touch

A half-century after the development of the first TVSS technologies, it is striking how infrequently they are used compared to other sensory aids or more technological advances in other fields. Economic and ergonomic factors have obviously played a large part in the marginal status of TVSS. The relatively high cost (around $10,000 for the 'lollipop' BrainPort™ TDU) explains its take-up for rehabilitation chiefly by the military, and will accelerate the further miniaturisation and ergonomic enhancement of the technology to make future iterations of the 'lollipop' increasingly wearable. Quite apart from these economic factors, another reason why TVSS may not enjoy more widespread uptake is because it simply cannot approach the performance of natural vision, in terms of the difference in density of nerve endings in the retina versus the tongue, and also the inability to perform saccade-like actions through tactile means. If the performance of TVSS is restricted by the nature of the sensory systems involved, therefore, it cannot be that these modalities are ultimately interchangeable and infinitely plastic. Instead, there are areas of functional equivalence within sensory subsystems, revealing forms of neuroplasticity that emerge through demonstrations of TVSS but also equally by other processes such as perceptual learning, sensory loss, sensory deprivation, and Braille reading. To be clear, TVSS does not directly attempt to re-engineer the touch system, creating an artificial modality. Rather, it simply transduces optical information into a format accessible to touch. The properties of the tactile system are then modified in ways described in this chapter, but only as a result of physiological response to the new kind of stimulation.

While it is conceivable in theory that certain technological manipulations might result in particular sensory modalities being interchangeable, at present this result cannot be achieved exclusively through the straightforward mechanism of the stimulation of one modality with information associated with another, that is, sensory substitution technology as it currently stands. This is due to the limitations of physiological plasticity, as we saw. Ultimately, the experimentally observed phenomenon of neuroplasticity does not in itself suggest a positive answer to the Molyneux question, or suggest any more general theory of an interchangeability of the senses, either. What sensory substitution devices offer, TVSS in particular, is something intriguing, bringing forth more touch-like forms of vision, or vision-like forms of touch, something extremely promising for congenitally and adventitiously blind subjects, especially those experiencing sudden blindness through injury.

Chapter 8

Blindness, Empathy, and 'Feeling Seeing': Literary Accounts of Blind Experience

Blindness is not darkness

Although Jorge Luis Borges rarely articulated his experiences as a blind man, he marked out what he called the 'pathetic moment' in 1955 when, for the purposes of both reading and writing, he became blind. Far from sudden, in his essay 'Blindness' he claims this occurred as a 'slow nightfall' (1999a: 474) that allowed him time to reflect upon the irreversibility of his descent into darkness. In other words, Borges, when sighted, anticipated that irreversible dread rift in experience, his impending blindness. For the sighted reader, the blind subject often prompts complex and attendant empathic responses. But following Smith's (1995) distinction, as sighted readers how do we feel *for*, or *with*, a subject who is, like Borges, countenancing a blindness yet to come? This chapter critically examines the fascination with blindness, with its asymmetry of curiosity, the allure of articulations of blind experience by blind writers. Is the mechanism one of sympathy, the sharing of the feelings of another (feeling-*with*), or the more specific projective identification of putting oneself in the place of another, empathy (feeling-*for*)? Through autobiographical writing, 'insider' accounts of blindness or impending blindness, and biographical fragments, the 'pathetic moment' recurs in some form through a number of authors and timelines, from Homer to Helen Keller, via Sophocles, Cicero, Milton, and Borges, to the self-styled 'Blind Traveller' James Holman.

One argument for the pervasiveness of the trope is that empathy, rather than sympathy, is the primary mechanism at stake. As Knight says of empathy within fiction, 'the sort of understanding we want to achieve involves us in the imaginative reduplication of how things are for someone else', and so authors 'employ the same folk psychology we use to understand and interpret the actions of others around us' (2006: 272). But as readers of autobiographical accounts of blindness and becoming-blind, what kinds of empathic responses are produced? Rather than mere reduplication, it could be argued, any act of reading involves an asymmetric curiosity. Furthermore, if readers of fictional or autobiographical accounts of blindness and of becoming-blind are themselves sighted, does the inherent asymmetry not become heightened, almost to the point of salaciousness? Given this asymmetry, what kind of empathic mechanism is involved in first anticipating, and then coming to terms with, the sighted reader's anxious imaginary of blindness as an irreversible, unremitting darkness? If sighted readers see blindness and the process of becoming-blind as a projection of their own fears, we might question the nature of their empathic response. We might, for instance, follow Garland-Thomson's investigation of disability in popular photography, 'The politics of staring', where the encounter with images of the disabled body is fraught with 'a tangle of distance, anxiety and identification' (2002: 57). Yet blindness and the process of becoming-blind fabricate their own interests and anxieties about sight loss, distinct from more corporeal concerns of physical disability. That tangle of distance and identification makes for an uneasy empathic relation, suffused as it is with fear and anxiety around the vulnerability of the eyes and the fragile mechanism of sight.

Our story of blindness, vision, and touch so far has only tangentially dealt with emotion or empathy. The newly sighted subjects who retreated from the visual world into the familiarity of darkness and touch, surveyed by Valvo (1971) and exemplified in Gregory and Wallace's (1963) case study 'S.B.', outwardly exhibited signs of depression but rarely articulated their internal affective states in their own words. This chapter redresses that paucity. For the sighted reader there is a duality of feeling, for alongside an enduring fascination with blindness and what the blind 'see' (e.g. Sacks 2003; Paterson 2006a; 2006b), a fascination that encompassed philosophical speculations and early psychological inquiry, early ophthalmic interventions, and public interest in narratives of recovery from blindness, arises an attendant inquisitiveness concerning what the blind *feel*. This latter aspect is manifested in two ways. First, in terms of literal feeling, the way the hands become more prominent, revealing a heightened tactile acuity in spatial perception and interaction. This is especially pronounced in movement and travelling, with the so-called 'Blind Traveller' James Holman writing a rich multisensory prose in his travelogue that foregrounds the haptic and the auditory.

Secondly, and more significantly for this chapter, there is a metaphorical feeling or an empathic feeling-with by the sighted reader of non-sighted experience, whether as temporary allegorical affliction such as Homer's treatment of Agamemnon in the *Iliad* ('blind rage', a period of unreason), or as irreversible medical condition. The well-worn tropes of the blind figure within literature are revisited through later biography and autobiography of blind subjects, deploying recognisable techniques or styles that prompt complex and provocative empathic responses on behalf of the blind by the sighted.

Whatever imaginary of blindness and sight loss the sighted entertain, it is important not to equate blindness with darkness. For example, José Luis Borges clearly dispels this assumption when describing the onset of full blindness: 'The world of the blind is not the night that people imagine' (1999a: 474). What sighted people imagine, however, remains irrevocably entwined with darkness, as we shall see throughout this chapter, an asymmetrical non-duplication of experience that forms a potentially misplaced cornerstone for readerly empathy. Does this association of blindness and darkness persist because of the limitations of language, the inability to find alternative metaphors that work so effectively for a sighted readership? Or is there a rhetorical necessity on the part of the author to communicate something of the strength of anxiety in the face of impending blindness?

While no sustained psychoanalytic approach is taken here, it is worth noting that Freud's references to the dramatically violent eye-gouging of Sophocles' *Oedipus the King* (c.429 BC) occur in various forms within his writings from 1897 right up to 1938. Why this continued fascination for Freud? The fear of blindness is primal and perennial and, unsurprisingly for Freud, one explanation for its origin lies in infantile sexuality. 'Concerning the factors of silence, solitude and darkness,' proclaims Freud in 'The Uncanny', 'we can only say that they are actually elements in the production of the infantile anxiety from which the majority of human beings have never become quite free' (1985: 376). Quite apart from associating blindness with castration, his allusion to the anxiety of the supposed isolating darkness of sightlessness is recognisable, and the persistent fascination with accounts of the blind and their embodied, spatial encounters are somewhat offset by their abject status. Applying Freud's ideas about the uncanny to disability and disease, for example, the geographer Wilton follows Garland-Thomson's formulation in *Extraordinary Bodies* (1997) by identifying those seen as having a physical disability as having 'incomplete or extraordinary bodies', and along with this the desire for abjection, 'to reject those things which are part of the body politic, but which generate anxiety' (Wilton, in Hubbard 2002: 122). Although Wilton is writing about AIDS sufferers in Los Angeles, and Garland-Thomson about representations of physical disabilities in American culture, the absence of functioning eyes renders those without sight similarly incomplete, extraordinary, and a source of anxiety for the sighted, in line with blind authors such as Hull (2001) or disability theorists like Michalko (1998; 2002).

The structure of this chapter is twofold. The first section, 'Feeling seeing', clarifies what definitions of blindness and empathy are being employed throughout, something of their genealogy, and introduces the methodological approaches applied to the literary texts. In the second section, 'Becoming-blind', I discuss three common tropes of blindness, devices employed to articulate some of the emotional resonances around impending, and actual, blindness. These include the anxieties of coming to terms with encroaching and irreversible blindness, the common but erroneous identification of blindness with darkness, the realisation of the consolations of blindness and the pleasures of touch, and the near-phenomenological rich description of becoming-blind, the actual process of losing sight. These are articulated in biography and autobiography at various historical points and through different writing positions and styles. At times the search for expression of blind experience relies on self-written 'insider accounts' (Davidson and Smith 2009: 903) that utilise introspective means (*specere* being Latin for 'looking', or 'to look at', implying inner vision). At other times the rich imaginary world is only incidentally a blind world. Before that, the character of feeling and empathy involved in texts that articulate experiences of blindness will be briefly examined.

Feeling seeing: a note on empathy, method, and meaning in blindness[1]

Theodor Lipps first used the word *Einfühlung* in his book on imitation in 1903. Having read this, and Lipps's essay on humour of 1905, Freud used the concept of *Einfühlung* to mean that 'we take the producing person's psychical state into consideration, put ourselves into it and try to understand it by comparing it with our own' (1960: 186). But whereas Freud later developed the concept

---

[1] 'Feeling seeing', the title of the article and indeed of this section, is an allusion to W. J. T. Mitchell's (2002) essay 'Showing seeing: a critique of visual culture'.

into an account of contemplating in others what is foreign to our own ego (see Wispé 1990: 21), the deployment of the term closest to Titchener's translation as 'empathy' (1908) is provided by June Downey, who summarises empathy as 'a process of "feeling-in" in which motor and emotional attitudes, however originating, are projected outside of the self' (1929: 176). Both somatic (motor) and affective (emotional) aspects will become significant later when examining descriptions of bodily movement, navigation, and travelogues of blind subjects. But Downey claims that our understanding of others is typically moulded by empathic processes: 'Through subtle imitation we assume an alien personality, we become aware of how it feels to behave thus and so, then we read back into the other person our consciousness of what [their] patterns of behaviour feel like' (1929: 177). Even as she wrote in 1929, Downey saw the term was already shifting according to different academic applications and contexts, but the core idea of projection of self-experiences into, or indeed on to, another person or thing remained (Wispé 1990: 34). Crucially, and unlike the strict definition of sympathy, empathy therefore allows the reader to retain their frame of reference while understanding the difference from another.

Quinodoz likewise in her *Words That Touch* defines empathy as a 'benevolent form of projective identification' which is 'a normal component of our day-to-day interactions' (2003: 108). In what follows, I take up this idea of empathy as 'projective identification' to examine the shifting relationships between sighted reader and non-sighted author according to three modes or authorial articulations of blind experience. The first relates to anxieties about impending blindness; the second to a shift from visual to non-visual, especially haptic, bodily experiences; and the third to the actual occurrence of blindness, the Borgesian 'pathetic moment'. Each case is drawn from experiential testimony, yet each charts different contours in the relationship between sighted and non-sighted, complicating the notion of empathy as a straightforward form of 'benevolent' identification, and returning in part to Titchener's emphasis on the role of a sensory imagination that includes the kinaesthetic within the mechanism of projection; to 'feel oneself *into* a situation', as Titchener had it (1916: 198, original emphasis). Empathy as 'projective identification' lies at the heart of the relationship between sighted reader and non-sighted author, then, and is surely heightened in the case of anxieties about the approach of blindness in the sighted.

Becoming-blind: empathic articulations of blindness

Despite the earlier literary examples that overcode blindness with predominantly negative emotions, throughout the book we have seen how the blind subject was treated as a hypothetical or blank figure, upon whom the epistemological theories and assumptions of the sighted author were projected. Whether it be the unnamed blind man discussed in Descartes' *Dioptrique*, the hypothetical blind man invoked in the correspondence between John Locke and William Molyneux, or the unnamed 'blind man of Puiseaux' of Diderot's *Lettre sur les aveugles*, the blind figure involved within philosophical speculation is often anonymous, 'the Hypothetical Blind Man' used as 'a prop for theories of consciousness' (Kleege 2005: 180). However, at various historical junctures the blind voice does get articulated, and these interspersed lone voices build into a chorus towards the twentieth century, when a number of highly personal and affecting autobiographical accounts of blindness and the process of becoming blind were offered. These voices include Helen Keller's *The Story of My Life* (1903) and *The World I Live In* (1908), which portray the inner world of a deaf-blind girl. Towards the end of that century, writings such as John Hull's account (1991) of descending into 'deep' blindness, Bryan Magee and Martin Milligan's philosophical exchange of letters (1998), literary theorist Georgina Kleege's account of macular degeneration (1999), blind sociologist Rod Michalko's work on blindness and disability studies (1998; 2002), and most recently Oliver Sacks's autobiographical account of vision impairment through ocular cancer (2010), all draw heavily upon first-person experiences. How do such first-person experiential accounts of blindness differ from the types of questionable testimonies that Cheselden reported after surgery in 1728, or that Diderot had invoked in the *Lettre*?

Anxiety in the face of darkness: Kleege and Hull

In a chapter on darkness in poetry, the sighted Susan Stewart asks this rhetorical question of her sighted reader: 'What do we fear when, in solitude, we fear absolute darkness?' It is not fear of death as such. 'In the end,' she surmises, 'the fear of darkness is the fear that the darkness will not end' (2002: 1). Imaginations of blindness by the sighted might be characterised by this fear of darkness without end, but as the vision-impaired writer and academic Georgina Kleege (1999) recognised, blindness is not darkness. Borges similarly describes the onset of his blindness in unsentimental prose: 'The world of the blind is not the night that people imagine' (1999a: 474). However, the fear of encroaching darkness, if not literal, resonates through poetic parallel. Witten three years before his death, Milton's 1671 poem *Samson Agonistes* mentions 'heaven's prime decree' which is God's first command in Genesis, 'Let there be light'. To become blind, to enter the world of darkness, is accordingly to counter this lucentric diktat. The protagonist Samson shares something of Milton's own agonistic journey into the world of blindness, struggling with darkness, isolation, and doubt, having had his eyes forcibly removed as punishment. Milton's own gradual descent into blindness was the result of disease, consecrated in a poem of 1655, 'On His Blindness'.

Such an antagonistic reaction to the indubitable power and certainty of God's declaration of light in the order of creation ('let there be light') is something that encapsulates or informs other accounts of the descent into blindness, what Derrida in *Memoirs of the Blind* terms 'specular isolation' (1993: 40). The irreversible journey into darkness is an acknowledgement of powerlessness against the machinery of vast forces, God's will, a sense of irredeemable imprisonment powerfully conveyed to the reader through the voice of Samson:

> Which shall I first bewail,
> Thy bondage or lost sight,
> Prison within prison
> Inseparably dark? Thou art become (O worst imprisonment)
> The dungeon of thyself. (*Samson Agonistes*, 151–6)

Anticipating his impending blindness in this way, does this not reflect the persistent dread fear and anxiety of blindness as darkness on the part of the sighted, and consequently further their inaccurate imaginary of blindness? The sense of the powerlessness of the protagonist is heightened by such dark imagery.

A far more recent and candid exchange of letters between philosophers directly questions this imaginary of blindness. The blind philosopher Martin Milligan accuses the sighted philosopher Bryan Magee of voicing the commonly held but prejudiced belief in an unbridgeable gulf between the experience of the sighted and of the blind, that vision constitutes a fundamental aspect of human existence and is therefore manifestly hungered for by the blind. For Milligan the blind philosopher, this assumption of a divide between the worlds of sight and of blindness is dangerously incorrect, effectively being 'sightist' or 'visionist'. He simply refuses to be cast into the assumed isolating darkness of solitude by the sighted Magee. Wilfully conflating the supposed actual blindness of darkness with the pejorative metaphor of blindness as ignorance for rhetorical effect, Milligan at one point betrays his exasperation. The blind Milligan argues that Magee's sightist statements concerning the appetite for vision seem

> to express the passion, the zeal of a missionary preaching to the heathen in outer darkness. Only [...] the message seems to be that ours is a 'darkness' from which we can never come in – not the darkness of course that sighted people can know, but the darkness of never being able to know that darkness, or of bridging the vast gulf that separates us from those who do. (Magee and Milligan 1998: 46)

Such exasperation is shared by other blind writers. *Sight Unseen*, Kleege's memoir of her descent into blindness, shows almost comically reflexive awareness of the tropes and conventions that autobiographies of blindness commonly exhibit. She scornfully characterises those authors as 'whiners' who declare that 'blindness is the worst disaster than can befall a human being', and dismisses the so-called 'blind mystics' who maintain 'the ancient myth of compensatory powers' and who 'wished to inspire awe in sighted readers with their coy allusions to second sight and extrasensory perception' (Kleege 1999: 3). There are exceptions, of course. Kleege's autobiographical writing is an example of the exercise of a critical inquisitiveness into the meaning and the experience of being 'blind', confronting some complex emotions involved in facing up to an impending, inevitable, and irreversible loss. Kleege's phenomenologically inclined reflections on the experience of her own low vision are examined in relation to the deaf-blind Helen Keller, below.

Autobiographical accounts of blindness sometimes directly address this heroic yet unwinnable struggle against the imagined onset of darkness, the blind theologian John Hull's *Touching the Rock* (1991) providing an almost paradigmatic example. In the early stages of sight loss Hull anticipates the inevitable loss of control that a continued descent into blindness entails by thinking in terms of dream imagery and, at least initially, in melodramatic terms of the struggle for control between light and darkness. Daily, small steps are taken, careful planning must be made. Otherwise, he says, 'I will have a sense of pointless desolation, a feeling of being carried helplessly deeper and deeper into it [the darkness]. The sense of subterranean or subconscious weight oppresses me, and I link in my mind the dream image of [a] huge, water-soaked hulk being dragged down into the depths' (1991: 39). Years later, reflecting back upon what resolved into distinct successive stages of blindness, each is characterised in emotional terms. The initial stage was preoccupied with hope, as he underwent a series of ultimately fruitless operations to rectify his condition. The occasional flickering of colour and light he experienced was quite possibly Charles Bonnet syndrome, when the overactive visual cortex compensates for the lack of visual stimulus as Sacks describes in *The Mind's Eye* (2010: 232). These dying echoes of visual activity, along with offers of help from faith healers, kept his hope alive. This passes, and the second stage is characterised by the business of overcoming the anticipated problems that his total blindness will bring, a feeling of readiness and expectation, purchasing and familiarising himself with assorted equipment and aids for vision impairment. Approximately a year afterwards, the third stage is characterised by anxieties about darkness which governed the majority of his waking life at the time, his routines and even his dreams. The fourth and final stage he describes as letting the blindness 'engulf' him (1991: 139), revealing an acclimatisation to his sightless condition combined with an element of fatalistic acceptance. Hull begins to ask whether during this stage of his journey into deep blindness, his closeness to God and the ability to muse theologically without the distractions of sight is actually a gift, albeit a 'dark, paradoxical gift' (1991: 155).

In considering blindness as a gift, we might consider the strangeness of a gift that the recipient cannot refuse, give back, defer; a gift that, like death, one has no choice but to accept, where the capacities of sight become devolved from the organs or particular body parts, instead diffusing and spreading throughout the body. Instead of seeing with the eyes, Hull describes in quasi-phenomenological terms a slow transformation towards seeing with the entire body, 'deep' blindness. Sensory pathways are reconfigured through the body, detecting objects in space through acoustic information (1991: 61), and the touch of the hand combined with internal bodily sensations including the feet (1991: 104). This process continues, in the absence of retinal stimulation. His perception becomes more haptocentric, involving heightened tactile and acoustic acuity and attunement to the somatosensory system (including balance, kinaesthesia, and proprioception). In a beautifully illustrative passage, woken by rainfall outside, Hull describes an enhanced sensory-spatial awareness as it is felt through the body:

> Is it true that the blind live in their bodies rather than in the world? I am aware of my body just as I am aware of the rain. My body is similarly made up of many patterns, many different regularities and irregularities, extended in space from down there to up here. These dimensions and details reveal themselves more and more as I concentrate my attention upon them. Nothing corresponds visually to this realization. Instead of having an image of my body, as being in what we call the 'human form,' I apprehend it now as these arrangements of sensitivities, a conscious space comparable to the patterns of the falling rain. The patterns of water envelope me in myriads of spots of awareness, and my own body is presented to me in the same way. There is a central area, of which I am barely conscious, and that seems to come and go. At the extremities, sensations fade into unconsciousness. My body and the rain intermingle, and become one audio-tactile, three-dimensional universe, within which and throughout the whole of which lies my awareness. (1991: 100)

At this point he explains his thought process as like a series of train carriages proceeding one after the other, a single-track line of consecutive speech, and receding into memory, forming part of an expanded three-dimensional awareness of the body as patterns of consciousness co-constituted by the rain and the body. But rain passes by, is fleeting: 'If the rain were to stop and I remain motionless here, there would be silence. My awareness of the world would again shrink to the extremities of my skin' (1991: 100).

Besides the myth of prophetic vision, another compensatory mechanism attributed to the blind by the sighted is heightened tactile sensitivity and auditory discrimination. There is a wealth of experimental neurological evidence for this (e.g. Goldreich and Kanics 2003; Röder and Rösler 2004). The ability to hear sounds at greater distances enhances spatial perception, bringing unseen objects or obstacles to awareness, while an increase in tactility is usually interpreted in terms of sensuous pleasure. Yet as his intensified awareness of the centrality of the body in spatial perception takes prominence, without visual distractions Hull feels drawn ever closer to God, a simultaneously spiritual and sensory reconfiguration. The dovetailing of abstract spirituality and the intensification of the sensory body in the last stage of his blindness leads to his becoming, in almost messianic terms, a self-described 'whole body seer' (1991: 164). For Hull, whole body seeing is not the gift of prophetic vision as in the case of Tiresias, but haptocentric perception, a heightening of non-visual perception, a rather different but more neurophysiologically constituted form of seeing feelingly, or seeing through the body. 'Increasingly, I do not think of myself so much as a blind person, which would define me with reference to sighted people and as lacking something, but simply as a whole-body seer', he reflects. 'A blind person is simply someone in whom the specialist function of sight is now devolved upon the whole body, and no longer specialized in a particular organ. Being a [whole body seer] is to be in one of the concentrated human conditions' (1991: 164). An undeniable clarity to his non-visual perceptions accompanies an appreciation of the tactile beauty of objects, and a renewed pleasure in the touching, feeling body. This is in common with other blind writers. There is a clarity to non-visual perceptions not because of his sightlessness, then, but due to the decoupling of 'seeing' from the eye, the organ of sight. For him this entails an appreciation of the positive aspects of non-visual experience such as the tactile beauty of objects and a renewed pleasure in the body. Such non-visual perceptions through the body will find comparable articulations in the two blind figures in the next sections.

The consolations and pleasures of touch: Cicero

If forging empathic understanding through writing is the goal in communicating experiences of blindness, there are also notable lacunae. In terms of discussions of pleasure, passions, the emotions, or even touch, it would seem that Stoic philosophy would be unfertile ground. However, around 45 BC at his villa in Tusculum, south-east of Rome, having studied Hellenistic philosophical sources, Cicero wrote in the form of the *consolatio*, a therapeutic text designed to ameliorate the aggravated passions of grief or sorrow (Erskin 1997). These texts became *Tusculan Disputations*, and in Book V, 'On virtue', he briefly summarises the dysfunctional role of the senses in pursuing a virtuous life. From Epicurus, Cicero considers the role of the senses in constituting pleasure. Can a wise man still be happy, asks Cicero, even if he is blind or deaf? Cicero evinces an astonishing lack of empathy in writing about blindness. The calamity that befalls anyone who has lost the use of their eyes is a 'dreadful thing', for which they must be consoled, hypothesises Cicero. He asks:

> What are the pleasures of which we are deprived by that dreadful thing, blindness? For though they allow other pleasures to be confined to the senses, yet the things which are perceived by the sight

do not depend wholly on the pleasure the eyes receive; as is the case when we taste, smell, touch or hear; for in respect of all these senses, the organs themselves are the seat of pleasure; but it is not so with the eyes. (2006: 469)

Even if little pleasure is derived from the eyes themselves, the legally blind disability theorist Rod Michalko has enough residual vision to 'pass' as sighted. He also returns to Cicero to reflect upon how the sighted have imagined blindness as lack, expressing consternation that this remains essentially true over two millennia later (1998: 141). Cicero's argument centres around the pleasures of the senses rather than their physiological function, suggesting that our imaginations and pleasures need not be solely visual. Even when visual, those pleasures are not situated in the organs of sight themselves. Again, invoking two common tropes of blindness, first in terms of darkness or night, and secondly that it is the mind which sees, rather than the eyes, Cicero continues:

For it is the mind which is entertained by what we see; but the mind may be entertained in many ways, even though we could not see at all. I am speaking of a learned and wise man, with whom to think is to live. But thinking in the case of the wise man does not altogether require the use of his eyes in his investigations; *for if night does not strip him of his happiness, why should blindness, which resembles night, have that effect?* (2006: 469–70, emphasis added)

Are we not dealing here with another Hypothetical Blind Man? Relying on prior Hellenistic philosophy and other secondary sources, Cicero quotes the blind Antipater of Cyrene, encapsulating the above sentiments through the allusion to the bodily and especially tactile pleasures one can feel even in darkness. Confronted by some women who bewailed his blindness, Antipater supposedly retorted: 'What do you mean? [...] do you think the night can furnish no pleasure?' (2006: 470). The heightening of sensuous tactility and intensification of embodied consciousness that Hull previously described also acknowledges a tension or Presocratic tendency that counters this, for the sighted Cicero or Diderot as for the blind Borges or Hull, leading from sensuality to cognitive abstraction. For, without the distractions of visual experience, another repeated trope is the ability to perform mathematical and geometrical abstractions.

Cicero relates apocryphal stories of blind philosophers, attributing special powers of abstraction to them including a heightened moral standing. Having little acquaintance with actual blind philosophers, in the case of Democritus of Abdera, the Atomist Presocratic philosopher, Cicero can only imaginatively infer that:

> Democritus was so blind he could not distinguish white from black: but he knew the difference betwixt good and evil, just and unjust, honourable and base, the useful and useless, great and small. Thus one may live happily without distinguishing colours; but without acquainting yourself with things, you cannot; and this man was of opinion, that the intense application of the mind was taken off by the objects that presented themselves to the eye, and while others often could not see what was before their feet, he travelled through all infinity. (2006: 471)

This same blind figure is referred to, much later, by Borges as having gouged out his own eyes in order to think more clearly. Borges identifies something of a perversity in this, or an admission of impotence, equating the act of eye-gouging once again, like Freud, with eviration, self-castration: 'Democritus of Abdera tore his eyes out in a garden so that the spectacle of reality would not distract him; Origen castrated himself' (1999a: 482). Since the word 'evirate' is an archaic form of self-castrate or emasculate, there is some crossover and association between the loss of orbis and loss of testes. Furthermore, both Cicero and Borges emphasise the metaphorical form of 'seeing' truth without eyes that persists within the sighted imaginary of blindness. This may in fact be the perfect encapsulation of the philosophical narrative of blindness prior to the twentieth century, a natural extension of Socrates' conceptualisation of vision as mental clarity and certitude as opposed to physical vision in Plato's *Symposium*, where the mind's eye grows critical even while the bodily eye fails: 'A man's mental vision does not begin to be keen until his physical vision is past its prime' (218d). Whether such a dramatic occurrence is historically verifiable or not, the significance of an unbounded intellect, the permanent truths of deep introspection as opposed to the fleeting visual distractions of the outside world, the ability to truly 'see' is unfettered by physiological uncertainties and therefore a more intuitive, noetic form of knowing. These are the kernels of the story of Democritus of Abdera. It is the perennial story of other mythic blind figures, as in Homer. And this apocryphal fragment persists in various forms, *mutatis mutandis*, for centuries. For example, Democritus' supposed non-physiological 'seeing' is repeated in an 1876 edition of *The Anatomy of Melancholy*, where Robert Burton compounds various fragments about Democritus alongside other blind figures to reach the same conclusion: 'Some philosophers and divines have evirated themselves, and put out their eyes voluntarily, the better to contemplate' (1876: 379).

Through the *consolatio*, the promise of non-visual and abstract pleasures for the sighted author promises consolation for any anticipated distress over sight loss, furthering that connection between *seeing* and *feeling* that is at the heart of the idea of empathic vision. For while as sighted readers we may feel pity or awe when faced with stories and accounts of blind subjects, even Cicero chides us for this unwarranted attribution. 'It is thus that the poets who represented Tiresias the Augur as a wise man and blind never exhibit him as bewailing his blindness', remarks Cicero (2006: 473). Nevertheless, just as Cicero, Burton, Borges, and others have alleged in their return to the Presocratics, blindness offers pleasures and gifts of its own, supposedly chief among which is the ability to contemplate, to pursue the inner mental life with greater clarity. For the Hypothetical Blind Man this would be a cognitive capacity, a clarity at the expense of clouded emotion. Is the attribution of such capacities to voiceless blind figures in fact contradicting, speaking against, the empathic writing suggested at the opening of this chapter?

Helen Keller's hand

We jump now from 45 BC to 1881, from Hypothetical Blind Man to actual embodied deaf-blind woman. As for others, the body and the hand plays a central part in navigating through darkness for Helen Keller. A disease at the age of eleven months robbed her of hearing as well as sight. In her more philosophically inclined and reflective passages, especially within *The World I Live In* (1908), Keller meditates on the hand, language, and sensory analogies, and provides what Kleege thinks is a 'detailed phenomenological account of her daily experience of deaf-blindness' (Kleege 2005: 184). Her introspective insights and sensory analogies certainly attempt to portray first-person fragments of deaf-blind experience to the reader. Naturally, this foregrounds the linguistic difficulties of transcribing such deaf-blind experience. Innocently enough, in one passage she writes 'I was taken to see a woman'. A footnote explains: 'The excellent proof-reader has put a query to my use of the word "see". If I had said "visit", he would have asked no questions, yet what does "visit" mean but to "see" (*visitare*)? Later I will try to defend myself for using as much of the English language as I have succeeded in learning' (Keller 2003: 19). Like any keen language learner and writer, her etymological knowledge escalates over time. Yet tellingly, the more comprehensive her understanding of etymological derivations is, the more difficult it is to find vocabulary without roots in either visual or auditory experience.

A significant autobiographical fragment concerns the hand. She conceptualises the hand as a 'pivot' through which all else is understood. Being both deaf and blind, it is this prehensile organ that bridges her darkness and isolation, inducts her into worldly and oneiric encounter alike:

> All my comings and goings turn on the hand as a pivot. It is the hand that binds me into the world of men and women. The hand is my feeler with which I reach through isolation and darkness and seize every pleasure, every activity that my fingers encounter. With the dropping of a little word from another's hand into mine, a slight flutter of the fingers, began the intelligence, the joy, the fullness of my life. (2003: 10)

In her blindness and the imagination, not the memory, of colour she then declares: 'My world is built of touch-sensations, devoid of physical color and sound; but without color and sound it breathes and throbs with life' (2003: 11). Not only prehensile, intentional, reaching ahead, the hand functions like a crucible for sensory transformation, the translation from one sense modality to another. The caress of a fresh-smelling flower becomes analogous to the crisp taste of a fresh apple. This information feeds into her imaginations of colour and resonates, the process of sensory analogue being familiar to us. For her, with only three functioning senses, this is an important imaginative gateway beyond potential sensory isolation, establishing a purview outside ocular experience to make alternative comparisons between sensory modalities. 'Some analogies I draw between qualities in surface and vibration, taste and smell, are drawn by others between sight, hearing and touch', she conjectures (2003: 68).

Appearing at various points in her autobiographical descriptions of her disabilities, Helen's hand is a relatively straightforward prehensile organ. Surprisingly, little she writes strays far from the historical kinds of conceptions of blindness by the sighted discussed so far. A possible reason for this is that she devours the writings of her philosophical forebears, and rearticulates them through her own voice. For example, at one point she asserts: 'If I had made a man, I should certainly have put the brain and soul in his fingertips' (2003: 73), an almost word-for-word restatement of Diderot's observation in the *Lettre*: 'If ever a philosopher, blind and deaf from his birth, were to construct a man after the fashion of Descartes, I can assure you, madam, that he would put the seat of the soul at the fingers' ends, for thence the greater part of the sensations and all his knowledge are derived' (1916a: 87). Elsewhere there are intimations of an original approach to embodied consciousness through descriptions of the dispersed and fragmented nature of tactile experience without sight, and acoustics as vibration. For physical and physiological reasons she cannot force her touch to pervade all things, imaginatively or otherwise. At times, their partial and fragmented nature disperses them: 'only small objects or small portions of a surface, mere touch-signs, a chaos of things scattered at random, remain...' (2003: 71). The partial and discontinuous nature of a world revealed not through vision or sound but through touch and vibration, which invites the prehensile hand to actively mediate, intercalate or transpose, reveals the centrality of the hand. As Kant says, the hand is the 'outer brain of man' (in Merleau-Ponty 1992: 316): A hand-centred thought, scoping and feeling its way, connects and smoothes discrete and fragmented spaces. This is something that Derrida, through Jean-Luc Nancy, would take forward. Referring to a passage in Nancy's *Corpus*, Derrida points to a kind of 'local' or 'fractal' touch (Nancy, in Derrida 2005: 127), a composite of tactile fragments, for while haptic certainty for the blind would benefit from smooth lines and tactile continuity, rarely does this happen outside the familiar space of the home. In an almost throwaway remark early in her autobiographical account, Keller asks us to '[r]emember that you, dependent on your sight, do not realize how many things are tangible' (2003: 11). This might effectively be a mantra for the partial, local, or fractal touch articulated by both Hull and Keller, as we have seen.

The pathetic moment: Borges and the Blind Traveller

We now come full circle. The blind figure as both writer and reader comes together in that trope of the realisation of blindness as irreversible nightfall, the Borgesian 'pathetic moment' that started this chapter. Strangely enough, blindness does not feature as a focus of Borges's output: a short essay and a few poems, unusually little for a writer whose rich imagination could interrogate the concepts and paradoxes of sight and blindness more exhaustively. Borges's ophthalmic condition was hereditary, and the first of seven operations for cataracts began in 1927, so the onset of blindness was irrevocable. As detailed in his 'Autobiographical essay' (1973), the darkness gathered pace in his fifties. Elsewhere he describes this as a 'modest blindness', not the dramatic sudden loss of sight that occurs within tragedy, a 'slow nightfall' that unfolded gradually until what he terms the 'pathetic moment' in 1955, the loss of his writer's and reader's sight (Borges 1999a: 474). Just as for Kleege, the long, slow, irreversible progress into night is felt most profoundly, the pathos most acute for a writer when the pages are unreadable, letters and faces lost amidst the fog. In one of only two poems that address this tragic and irreversible process he says:

> Both days and nights would wear away the profiles
> Of human letters and of well-loved faces. ('The Blind Man' 1999b: 311)

Even so, he is characteristically philosophical. 'Blindness has not been for me a total misfortune', he later declares in his essay 'Blindness'. 'It should not be seen in a pathetic way. It should be seen as a way of life, one of the styles of living' (1999a: 478). Blindness as a way of life, rather than a pitiful condition; a remarkably affirmatory statement from a sighted perspective, but commonplace among blind and visually impaired writers like Helen Keller, John Hull, and Georgina Kleege.

But this is far from the epic struggle between darkness and light that characterises Milton's *Samson Agonistes*. In Milton, Borges finds a profound commonality with the ageing and blinded composer of verses, a poet whose memory had to adjust in proportion to the irreversible diminution of his visual world. Memorising piecemeal for visitors and guests, the whole of *Samson Agonistes* was written this way, the lyrical memory of a blind Homer once again. The commonality extends. In his 1655 sonnet 'On his Blindness', Milton describes something of his own identification of blindness and inner sinfulness and despair with the lines: 'When I consider how my light is spent/ Ere half my days, in this dark world and wide' (1866: 212). Borges refers to this passage, recognising this portrait of blindness, but as in Derrida's *Memoires sur l'aveugles* ['Memoirs of the blind'] (1993) connecting it to an apprehensive body, an anxious prehensile hand that constantly gropes ahead, actively seeking tactile reassurance: 'It is precisely the world of the blind when they are alone, walking with hands outstretched, searching for props', Borges explains from experience (1999a: 480). Considering the role of imagination and the writing process itself, Borges declares that the best of Milton's poetry was realised when blind, memorised and then dictated to his daughters and casual visitors.

As a blind writer reading the poetry and prose of other writers, Borges did not consider his own life as unfortunate. He quotes with approval James Joyce's declaration that 'of all the things that have happened to me, I think the least important was having been blind' (Borges 1999a: 481). Musing upon this, Borges allows himself a passing fantasy of Joyce at the writing desk, where much of his work was produced in near-darkness. If the reader is effectively blind, as Kleege has said, then the writing process is positively myopic, straining, focused, and repetitious, struggling to get it right. Not just for writers like Milton, who became totally blind and dictated his verse to sighted helpers, or Joyce, whose sight was literally failing, or Kleege who strains through all kinds of optical technologies to keep reading and writing on the very cusp of her macular degeneration. The following that was said of Joyce could equally be said of the writing process in general: 'Part of his vast work was executed in darkness: polishing the sentences in his memory, working for a whole day on a single phrase, and then writing it and correcting it. All in the midst of blindness or periods of blindness' (Borges 1999a: 481).

It is difficult not to be mindful of this when reading the notebooks of one celebrated blind figure of the early nineteenth century, James Holman RN, who also quotes Milton's poem, himself railing against 'heaven's prime decree' about light in his newfound darkness, undergoing his own pathetic moment yet only writing tangentially about it. Perhaps as a form of distancing from this traumatic period of adjustment to his blindness, and the sober and far-reaching realisation that his career in the Royal Navy was precipitously terminated, the young and then-promising Lieutenant Holman refers to himself in the third person briefly, and for the only time, in his journal:

> It is sufficient to say, that at the age of twenty-five [...] his prospects were irrevocably blighted by the effects of an illness, resulting from his professional duties, and which left him deprived of all the advantages of 'heaven's prime decree' – wholly – and, he fears, permanently blind. (Holman 1822: vi)

Like Borges, thereafter he rarely refers to his own blindness throughout his journals or bestselling published travelogues. For Holman's blindness in his twenties was no barrier to extensive travels, including a circumnavigation of the globe in that great period of exploration. Styling himself the 'Blind Traveller', Holman became a member of an exclusive dining circle known as the Raleigh Club, named after Sir Walter Raleigh, and later absorbed into the Royal Geographical

Society. The cause of his blindness was unknown during his lifetime but symptoms suggest uveitis, death of the optic nerve through the inflammation of the middle tissue of the eye, today the third-biggest cause of blindness in the United States after diabetes and macular degeneration (Suttorp-Schulten and Rothova 1996). Curiously, the more he travelled and wrote, the less reference he made to his blindness. In *A Voyage Round the World, Including Travels in Africa, Asia, Australasia, America etc. etc.* (1834), his blindness is mentioned only in the preface, pitched to the reader not as a handicap but as enabling him to be a superior investigator of novel cultures. Echoing the familiar wisdom of the Hypothetical Blind Man, and especially of that type of blindness that for Plato meant the freeing up of the mind's eye, Holman claimed in the *Voyage*: 'Freed from the hazard of being misled by appearances, I am the less likely to adopt hasty and erroneous conclusions.' 'I always vividly remember the daily occurrences which I wish to retain, so that it is not possible that any circumstances can escape my attention' (Holman 1834: 6).

As a blind figure, Holman instils a sense of boldness, initiative, and adventure, but also betrays an increasingly cultivated, non-visual, aesthetic sensibility towards the world. Sighted readers and biographers attribute to him literally an 'inner vision', albeit one attuned to the aesthetic, that earlier idea of 'feeling seeing', where the aesthetic deals not only with matters of taste but also etymologically with the feeling body (*aesthesis* for Aristotle being the sensory faculty; see e.g. Danius 2002). Towards the end of his life an American anthology recounts Holman's restless itineraries and captivity, and explains his appreciation of female beauty and musings on female charms despite his blindness. In his biographer's words, Holman showed an appreciation for 'the exquisite delight with which his inner vision drank in scenes of beauty' (Roberts 2006: 333). A particular episode in Holman's travelogues exemplifies such 'inner vision' as an aesthetic response, and remains neurologically elucidating despite his unwillingness to articulate his blindness directly in the travelogues. Shortly after his own 'pathetic moment', newly blind but with visual memories intact, one evening he attended the theatre. Despite his sightless state he reported the overwhelmingly convincing, almost overpowering experience of 'seeing' one of the actresses: 'The flood of sensation had begun to mingle and fuse, transforming into something entirely new. This was no mind's-eye mental image – it seemed tantamount to sight' (Roberts 2006: 333). Holman's published journal, written initially on carbonated paper through a Noctograph, a precursor to a Braille machine, records: 'I heard, I felt, I saw, or *imagined I saw*, everything which words, gestures and actions could convey' (1822: 129, his italics).

Charles Bonnet syndrome provides a medical explanation for phantom images in cases of recent blindness, as impulses in a still-functioning visual cortex would produce a form of exquisite synaesthesia for a blind man coming to terms with the condition (see e.g. Ramachandran and Blakeslee 1998: 85ff.). Yet the significance for Holman is that it *felt* as though he really saw, and sadness remains in the awakened sensory memory of what was now, for him, forever lost.

Like Hull and Keller, at some stage in his travelogues there is a distinct shift to the haptic, at first the roaming hand which apprehends and mediates, and subsequently a more somatocentric consciousness. Accordingly, we consider how the increasingly haptocentric Holman more artfully renders landscapes and scenes, given the absence of vision. The pictorial metaphors are apt, making evident a phase change in aesthetic appreciation of haptic qualities for Holman, pursuing his aesthetic sensibility increasingly through the hands and body. Whether the price of cologne in Cologne or the height of Rome's Tomb of Cestius, much was dutifully catalogued and recorded, his haptic explorations physically marked and inscribed through the Noctograph writing machine. 'The whole of his experience was still raw sense memory and haptic knowledge,' explains Roberts, 'ready to be fitted out with words and unloosed in a stream of narrative' (2006: 248).

Yet this stream of haptic narrative rendered into text for the sighted reader evokes a series of primarily visual encounters and landscapes. Once published, Holman's journals attracted the ire of critics who doubted the blind traveller's authenticity of encounter with a world he could never optically 'see', the predictable assumption being that certainty is ocular, that authenticity in 'being there' is confirmed through vision alone. This one question at the heart of the sighted experience of reading Holman recurs when he pointedly asks himself: 'What is the use of travelling to one who cannot see?', to which he replies:

> The picturesque in nature, it is true, is shut out from me, and works of art are to me mere outlines of beauty, accessible to only one sense; but perhaps this very circumstance affords a stronger zest to curiosity, which is thus impelled to a more close and searching examination of details than would be considered necessary to a traveller who might satisfy himself with the superficial view. (Holman 1834: 4)

Later he considers it an advantage that there is no purple prose romanticising his encounters, wrapping it in the fashionable language of the sublime and the picturesque, so that 'these magnificent sights do not make pages of pictures in my work' (1840: 5). In aesthetic appreciation of foreign lands and people, then, his blindness connotes no lack. Despite this sensorily-rich travel, or travel as generalised haptic sensibility or disposition towards the landscape and environment, fuller multisensory descriptions are attempted. At times he writes as he walks, by feeling his way. In a brief prefatory passage in a later travelogue, Holman writes almost plaintively about the difficulties of representing his blind experience, sensations of air pressure and wind taking increased prominence in his experience of landscape:

> On the summit of the precipice, and in the heart of the green woods [...] there was an intelligence in the winds of the hills, and in the solemn stillness of the buried foliage, that could not be mistaken. It entered into my heart, and I could have wept, *not that I did not see, but that I could not portray all that I felt.* (1840: 6, emphasis added)

That final sentence could work as a leitmotif for any traveller, blind or sighted. If Holman's haptic appreciation of objects also begins to extend to a more distributed cutaneous sensing of the environment through air pressure and acoustics, it becomes ever more difficult to evoke or describe such experience. His powers of description inevitably fall short. Yet prior to any more sustained psychological examination of the phenomenon of 'facial vision', where air pressure felt on the face for example indicates the proximity and spatial location of an object (see e.g. Hull 1991; Sacks 2010), Holman unsurprisingly articulates a more poetically haptocentric rendering of his experience and his environment and, like Keller's hand as a pivot, employs not only cross-modal sensations but also cross-modal metaphors, of feeling his seeing. Indeed, in the frontispiece to his 1840 volume *Travels in China, New Zealand, New South Wales, Van Diemen's Land, Cape Horn* he quotes from *King Lear*, where the character Gloucester has been forcibly blinded. Upon Lear remarking: 'You see how the world goes', Gloucester famously replies: 'I see it feelingly' (IV, iv).

Conclusion: life 'after' sight

Feeling seeing, or seeing feelingly returns us finally to the discussion of empathic vision, where the relation between blind writer and predominantly sighted reader is characterised by projective identification, a sharing of affective experience, motivated by an inquisitiveness about the experiences of a blind other. Literary tropes and persistent myths of blindness were counterbalanced by autobiographical or 'insider' accounts. To some extent empathic vision emplaces us, through such projective identification, to share the intensified pathos, the anxieties of darkness and becoming-blind, or conversely to share in the pleasures and consolations of touch. But equally, descriptions, portrayals, and evocations of aesthetic experience by a non-visual subject have heightened the role of the haptic, of somatic sensibilities, of the need to articulate non-visual experiences, through sensory associations and analogues, that indicate a sensorily reconfigured body, for Holman, Keller, and Hull alike.

The loaded language of loss or lack associated within the terms blindness or vision impairment perhaps too readily invokes or suggests its opposite. Against the constructed figure of the disabled body is what Garland-Thomson terms the 'normate body', replete in all its senses, both metaphorically and physiologically. The normate is, just like the blank-blind figure above, 'the constructed identity of those who, by way of the bodily configurations and cultural capital they assume, can step into a position of authority and wield the power it grants them' (1997: 8). Yet with the various impairments or positions on the spectrum of disability or age, the strength of the normate figure lies not in population or number. Rather, the figure of the normate has the potential to complicate positions that deal with cultural and physical 'otherness', doing so beyond any restrictive dichotomy, especially in this case of sighted/blind. Naomi Schor's analysis of metaphorical blindness within French literature and cinema, for example, similarly claims that the return to 'the body' in social theory at the end of the twentieth century, with its complex problematics of pains, pleasures, and significations, nonetheless betrayed the fact that 'the Body qua body has been posited as integral, as fully sensate' (1999: 84), and therefore in Garland-Thomson's terms, normate. Such background assumptions belong to the 'Empire of the Normal', as Kleege writes in an essay on Keller. Invoking the normate here holds a mirror up to the pervasive and compelling construction of the blind figure for a readership that encompasses the spectrum of complete blindness, vision impairment, or a sighted body, while inviting further consideration of any (a)symmetries of readerly empathy. Alongside Schor I have argued that rich metaphorical seams throughout history may fruitfully bear extensive analysis through manifestations in recurring tropes, blind figures or, following Kleege, Hypothetical Blind Men. Examining some of the pervasive tropes and characterisations of blind experience, by both sighted and blind, reveals associated emotions and anxieties about blindness as darkness, of the anxieties of loss of sight, but also of the pleasures, consolations, and compensations of touch and haptocentrism. But at one point in her analysis of metaphors Schor chimes: 'It is time to consider the body as the locus of sensory deprivation that is not reducible to metaphors, discourses, myths, and all manner of idealistic constructs, but that is not intelligible outside of language' (1999: 84).

In other words, reflections upon the many and variegated experiences of blindness and visual impairment reveal the task of explaining or exploring such experience through language as problematic, however well the tensions within metaphorical blindness are teased or unpicked. Is it not naive to posit, as Schor does, a reconceptualised body that might be attuned to a non-normate sensorium, one lacking the functionalities of particular sense(s), yet integrated in its own way through cross-modal perceptions, through creative use of sensory analogues? Furthermore, in facing up to and anticipating the pathetic moment, is there not 'a life after sight' which is detached from the nostalgia of vision and visual memory, as Bradford and Hull suggest (2011: 128)? As some of the surveyed blind figures attempted in their sometimes indirect or straining attempts to represent an under-represented seam of non-visual experiences, from Milton's solitary imprisonment in blindness, the sensory analogies and haptocentric world of Helen Keller, the whole body seeing and somatocentric perception of Hull, or the outwardly-facing haptic aesthetic engagements with the world of the 'Blind Traveller' James Holman, we can ask: Is there some seam of non-normate, non-replete experience which remains defined not in terms of sensory lack or loss, but which finds explanation through other, more somatocentric means? Is this perhaps the actual inception of sensory difference and explanation? For, on losing one's sight, one does not lose one's eyes, believes Marvell: 'Only then does man [sic] begin to *think* the eyes' (Derrida 1993: 128, original emphasis).

References

Abbott, T. K. (1864), *Sight and Touch: An Attempt to Disprove the Received (or Berkleian), Theory of Vision*, London: Longman.
Abbott, T. K. (1904), 'Fresh light on Molyneux's problem: Dr. Ramsay's case', *Mind* 13(52): 543–54.
Ackroyd, C., Humphrey, N. K., and Warrington, E. K. (1974), 'Lasting effects of early blindness: a case study', *Quarterly Journal of Experimental Psychology* 26: 114–24.
Addison, J. (1712), 'On the pleasures of the imagination', *The Spectator* 411–22: 593–609.
American Foundation for the Blind (2002), 'Living with low vision', http://www.afb.org/Section.asp?SectionID=26&TopicID=144 (accessed 19 October 2008)
Albert, D. M. (1997), 'Notes on Voltaire's "The Elements of Sir Isaac Newton's Philosophy"', *Documenta Ophthalmologica* 94: 59–81.
Anonymous (1784), 'Variétés, Aux auteurs du Journal', *Journal de Paris* 115, 24 April, 504–5. Available online from the 17th-18th Century Burney Collection of the British Library, http://www.bl.uk/reshelp/findhelprestype/news/newspdigproj/burney/ (accessed 18 January 2013).
Appelbaum, D. (1995), *The Stop*, Albany, NY: State University of New York Press.
Bach-y-Rita, P. (1972), *Brain Mechanisms in Sensory Substitution*, New York: Academic Press.
Bach-y-Rita, P., and Kercel, S. W. (2003), 'Sensory substitution and the human–machine interface', *Trends in Cognitive Sciences* 7: 541–6.
Bach-y-Rita, P., Collins, C. C., Saunders, F., White, B., and Scadden, L. (1969), 'Vision substitution by tactile image projection', *Nature* 221: 963–4.
Bach-y-Rita, P., Kaczmarek, K. A., et al. (1998), 'Form perception with a 49-point electrotactile stimulus array on the tongue', *Journal of Rehabilitation Research Development* 35: 427–30.
Baddely, A. D. (1992), 'Working memory', *Science* 255: 256–9.
Baker, H. F. (2007), 'Saunderson, Nicholas (bap. 1683, d. 1739)', rev. James J. Tattersall, *Oxford Dictionary of National Biography*, Oxford University Press, 2004; online edn, http: //www.oxforddnb.com/view/article/24709 (accessed 8 October 2012).

Barasch, M. (2001), *Blindness: The History of a Mental Image in Western Thought*, London: Routledge.
Bavelier, D., and Neville, H. (2002), 'Cross-modal plasticity: where and how?', *Nature Reviews Neuroscience* 3: 443–52.
Baxandall, M. (1997), *Shadows and Enlightenment*, New Haven, CT: Yale University Press.
Berkeley, G. (1975), *Philosophical Works, Including the Works on Vision*, ed. M. R. Ayers, London: Everyman.
Berkeley, G. (1996) [1709], *An Essay Towards a New Theory of Vision*, London, Everyman.
Bolt, D. (2003), 'Blindness and the problems of terminology', *Journal of Visual Impairment & Blindness* 97(9): 519–20.
Bolton, M. B. (1994), 'The real Molyneux problem and the basis of Locke's answer', in G. A. Rogers (ed.), *Locke's Philosophy: Content and Context*, Oxford: Oxford University Press, 75–99.
Borges, J. L. (1973), 'An autobiographical essay', in *The Aleph and Other Stories 1933–1969*, trans. N. T. di Giovanni, London: Pan Books.
Borges, J. L. (1999a), 'Blindness', in *Selected Non-Fictions*, ed. E. Weinburger, trans. E. Allen, S. J. Levine, and E. Weinburger, New York: Viking, 473–83.
Borges, J. L. (1999b), *Selected Poems*, ed. A. Coleman, New York: Viking.
Botvinick, M., and Cohen, J. (1998), 'Rubber hands "feel" touch that eyes see', *Nature* 391(6669): 756.
Bowcott, O. (2010), 'Device lets blind soldier "see" with his tongue', *The Guardian*, 16 March, 13.
Bowler, P. J. (2003), *Evolution: The History of an Idea*, Berkeley: University of California Press.
Bradford, D., and Hull, J. (2011), 'Another blinding documentary on Channel 4?', *Journal of Visual Culture* 10: 125–3.
Brewer, D. (2006), *The Discourse of Enlightenment in Eighteenth-Century France: Diderot and the Art of Philosophizing*, Cambridge: Cambridge University Press.
Bruno, M., and Mandelbaum, E. (2010), 'Locke's answer to Molyneux's thought experiment', *History of Philosophy Quarterly* 27(2): 165–80.
Bubic, A., Striem-Amit, E., et al. (2010), 'Large-scale brain plasticity following blindness and the use of sensory substitution devices', in M. J. Naumer and J. Kaiser (eds), *Multisensory Object Perception in the Primate Brain*, Berlin: Springer.
Büchel, C., et al. (1998), 'Different activation patterns in the visual cortex of late and congenitally blind subjects', *Brain* 121: 409–19.
Buffon, G. L. L. (1797) [1749], *Buffon's Natural History*, Vol. IV, trans. J. S. Barr, London: H. D. Symonds.
Burr, D. C., and Morrone, M. C. (2004), 'Visual perception during saccades', in J. S. Werner and L. M. Chalupa (eds), *The Visual Neurosciences*, Cambridge, MA: MIT Press, 1391–401.

Burton, R. (1876), *The Anatomy of Melancholy, What it is, its kinds, causes, symptoms, prognostics. And several cures of it*, London: William Tegg and Co.

Campbell, F. J. (1910), 'Blindness', *The Encyclopaedia Britannica*, 11th edition, Vol. IV, 59–72.

Candela, A. R. (2003), 'A rehabilitationist's notebook: Oliver Sacks on blindness', *The Braille Monitor* 46(10), nfb.org (accessed 22 May 2013).

Carreiras, M., and Codina, B. (1992), 'Spatial cognition of the blind and sighted – visual and amodal hypotheses', *Cahiers de psychologie cognitive–Current Psychology of Cognition* 12(1): 51–78.

Cassirer, E. (1979), *The Philosophy of the Enlightenment*, Princeton: Princeton University Press.

Cattaneo, Z., and Vecchi, T. (2011), *Blind Vision: The Neuroscience of Visual Impairment*, Cambridge, MA: MIT Press.

Cheselden, W. (1728), 'An account of some observations made by a young gentleman, who was born blind, or who lost his sight so early, that he had no remembrance of ever having seen, and was couch'd between 13 and 14 years of age', *Philosophical Transactions* 402: 447–50.

Chirimuuta, M., and Paterson, M. (2014), 'A methodological Molyneux question: sensory substitution, plasticity and the unification of perceptual theory', in D. Stokes, M. Matthen, and S. Biggs (eds), *Perception and its Modalities*, Oxford: Oxford University Press, 410–30.

Cicero (2006), *The Academic Questions, Treatise De Finibus and Tusculan Disputations of M. T. Cicero, With a Sketch of the Greek Philosophers Mentioned by Cicero*, trans. C. D. Yonge, Whitefish, MT: Kessinger Publishing.

Clark, S. (2007), *Vanities of the Eye: Vision in Early Modern European Culture*, Oxford: Oxford University Press.

Cohen, L. G., Celnik, P., et al. (1997), 'Functional relevance of cross-modal plasticity in blind humans', *Nature* 389: 180–3.

Condillac, E. B. (1930) [1754], *Condillac's Treatise on the Sensations*, trans. G. Carr, Los Angeles: University of Southern California Press.

Condillac, E. B. (1982), *Philosophical Writings of Etienne Bonnot, Abbé de Condillac*, trans. F. Philip, Mahwah, NJ: Lawrence Erlbaum Associates.

Crary, J. (1990), *Techniques of the Observer: On Vision and Modernity in the Nineteenth Century*, Cambridge, MA: MIT Press.

Crary, J. (1999), *Suspensions of Perception: Attention, Spectacle, and Modern Culture*, Cambridge, MA: MIT Press.

Creech, J. (1986), *Diderot: Thresholds of Representation*, Columbus, OH: Ohio State University Press.

Cru, R. L. (1913), *Diderot as a Disciple of English Thought*, New York: Columbia University Press.

Curran, A. (2000), 'Diderot's revisionism: enlightenment and blindness in the "Lettre sur les aveugles"', *Diderot Studies* 28: 75–93.

D'Alembert, J. L. R. (1772), 'Blindness', in *Selected Essays from the Enclyopedy*, London: Samuel Leacroft, 132–47.

Danius, S. (2002), *The Senses of Modernism: Technology, Perception and Aesthetics*, Ithaca, NY: Cornell University Press.

Davidson J., and Smith, M. (2009), 'Autistic autobiographies and more-than-human emotional geographies', *Environment and Planning D: Society and Space* 27(5): 898–916.

Davis, J. W. (1960), 'The Molyneux problem', *Journal of the History of Ideas* 21(3): 392–408.

De Fontenay, E. (1982), *Diderot: Reason and Resonance*, trans. Jeffrey Mehlman, New York: George Braziller.

De La Sizeranne, F. (1894), *The Blind as Seen Through Blind Eyes*, trans. F. P. Lewis, London: G. P. Putnam's Sons.

Degenaar, M. (1996), *Molyneux's Problem: Three Centuries of Discussion on the Perception of Forms*, trans. M. J. Collins, London: Kluwer Academic Publishers.

Deroy, O., and Auvray, M. (2014), 'A crossmodal perspective on sensory substitution', in D. Stokes, M. Matthen, and S. Biggs (eds), *Perception and its Modalities*, Oxford: Oxford University Press, 327–48.

Derrida, J. (1993), *Memoirs of the Blind: The Self Portrait and Other Ruins*, trans. Pascale-Anne Brault and Michael Naas, Chicago: University of Chicago Press.

Derrida, J. (2005), *On Touching – Jean-Luc Nancy*, trans. C. Irizarry, Stanford: Stanford University Press.

Descartes, R. (1965), *Discourse on Method; Optics; Geometry; and Meteorology*, trans. J. Olcamp, New York: Library of the Liberal Arts.

Descartes, R. (1985), *The Philosophical Writings of Descartes*, trans. J. Cottingham, R. Stoothoff, and D. Murdoch, Cambridge: Cambridge University Press.

Descartes, R. (1995) [1641], *Discourse on Method and the Meditations*, trans. F. E. Sutcliffe, Harmondsworth: Penguin.

Descartes, R. (2001) [1637], 'Optics', in *Discourse on Method, Optics, Geometry, and Meteorology*, trans. P. J. Olscamp, Indianapolis: Hackett Publishing.

Descartes, R. (2003) [1664], *Treatise of Man*, trans. T. S. Hall, Amherst, NY: Prometheus Books.

Descartes, R. (2008) [1641], *Meditations on First Philosophy with Selections from the Objections and Replies*, trans. M. Moriarty, Oxford: Oxford University Press.

Diderot, D. (1916a) [1749], 'Letter on the blind', in M. Jourdain (ed.), *Diderot's Early Philosophical Works*, Chicago: Open Court Publishing.

Diderot, D. (1916b) [1782], 'Addition to the preceding letter', in M. Jourdain (ed.), *Diderot's Early Philosophical Works*, Chicago: Open Court Publishing.

Diderot, D. (2000) [1754], *Thoughts on the Interpretation of Nature and Other Philosophical Works*, trans. L. Sandler, London: Clinamen Press.

Doidge, N. (2007), *The Brain That Changes Itself: Stories of Personal Triumph from the Frontiers of Brain Science*, Harmondsworth: Penguin.
Downey, J. E. (1929). 'A few words on empathy', in *Creative Imagination: Studies in the Psychology of Literature*, New York: Harcourt Brace, 175–8.
Edgell, B. (1932), 'Current constructive theories in psychology', British Association for the Advancement of Science Report, London: Burlington House, 169–84.
Eilan, N. (1993), 'Molyneux's question and the idea of an external world', in N. Eilan, R. McCarthy, and B. Brewer (eds), *Spatial Representation: Problems in Philosophy and Psychology*, Oxford: Blackwell, 236–55.
Erskin, A. (1997), 'Cicero and the expression of grief', in S. M. Braund and C. Gill (eds), *The Passions in Roman Thought and Literature*, Cambridge: Cambridge University Press, 36–47.
Evans, G. (1985), 'Molyneux's question', in *Gareth Evans: Collected Papers*, ed. A. Phillips, Oxford: Clarendon Press.
Farrell, G. (1956), *The Story of Blindness*, Cambridge, MA: Harvard University Press.
Feeney, D. (2007), *Toward an Aesthetics of Blindness: An Interdisciplinary Response to Synge, Yeats, and Friel*, New York: Peter Lang.
Findlay, J. M., and Gilchrist, I. D. (2003), *Active Vision: The Psychology of Looking and Seeing*, Oxford: Oxford University Press.
Fine, I. (2009), 'Recovery of vision following blindness', in E. Bruce Goldstein (ed.), *Encyclopedia of Perception*, Thousand Oaks, CA: Sage, 865–8.
Fine, I., Wade, A., Boynton, G. M. B., Brewer, A., May, M., Wandell, B., et al. (2003), 'The neural and functional effects of long-term visual deprivation on human cortex', *Nature Neuroscience* 6: 915–16.
Finger, S. (1994), *Origins of Neuroscience: A History of Explorations into Brain Function*, Oxford: Oxford University Press.
Fischer, B., and H. Weber (1993), 'Express saccades and visual attention', *Behavioral and Brain Sciences* 16: 553–610.
Foucault, M. (1973) [1966], *The Order of Things: An Archaeology of the Human Sciences*, New York: Vintage.
Foucault, M. (2002) [1969], *The Archaeology of Knowledge*, trans. A. M. Sheridan Smith, London: Routledge.
Foucault, M. (2003) [1963], *The Birth of the Clinic: An Archaeology of Medical Perception*, trans. A. M. Sheridan Smith, London: Routledge.
Franz, J. C. A. (1839), *A Treatise on the Art of Preserving the Eye, &c. &c.*, London: J. Churchill.
Freud, S. (1960) [1905], *Jokes and their Relation to the Unconscious*, trans. J. Strachey, New York: W.W. Norton.
Freud, S. (1985) [1919], 'The Uncanny', in *Pelican Freud Library*, Vol. 14, trans. J. Strachey, Harmondsworth: Penguin.
Friel, B. (1994), *Molly Sweeney, A Play*, Harmondsworth: Penguin.
Gallagher, S. (2005), *How The Body Shapes the Mind*, Oxford: Clarendon Press.

Ganson, T., and Ganson, D. (2010), 'Everyday thinking about bodily sensations', *Australasian Journal of Philosophy* 88(3): 523–34.

Garland-Thomson, R. (1997), *Extraordinary Bodies: Figuring Physical Disability in American Culture and Literature*, New York: Columbia University Press.

Garland-Thomson, R. (2002), 'The politics of staring: visual rhetorics of disability in popular photography', in S. L. Snyder, B. J. Brueggemann, and R. Garland-Thomson (eds), *Disability Studies: Enabling the Humanities*, New York: Modern Language Association of America, 56–75.

Gibson, J. J. (1950), *The Perception of the Visual World*, London: George Allen & Unwin.

Gibson, J. J. (1962), 'Observations on active touch', *Psychological Review* 69(6): 477–91.

Gibson, J. J. (1966), *The Senses Considered as Perceptual Systems*, Boston: Houghton Mifflin.

Gibson, J. J. (1979), *The Ecological Approach to Visual Perception*, Hillsdale, NJ: Lawrence Erlbaum Associates.

Gitter, E. (2001), *The Imprisoned Guest: Samuel Howe and Laura Bridgman, the Original Deaf-Blind Girl*, New York: Farrar, Straus, and Giroux.

Goldreich, D., and Kanics, I. M. (2003), 'Tactile acuity is enhanced in blindness', *Journal of Neuroscience* 23: 2445–3439.

Goldstein, J. (2003), 'Bringing the psyche into scientific focus', in T. M. Porter and D. Ross (eds), *The Cambridge History of Science, Vol. VII: The Modern Social Sciences*, Cambridge: Cambridge University Press, 131–53.

Graven, T. (2003), 'Aspects of object recognition: when touch replaces vision as the dominant sense modality', *Visual Impairment Research* 5(2): 101–12.

Grayling, A. C. (2005), *Descartes: The Life and Times of a Genius*, New York: Walker and Co.

Gregory, R. L. (1967), *Eye and Brain: The Psychology of Seeing*, London: World University Library.

Gregory, R. L. (2003), 'Seeing after blindness', *Nature Neuroscience* 6: 915–16.

Gregory, R. L. (2004), 'The blind leading the sighted: an eye-opening experience of the wonders of perception', *Nature* 430: 836.

Gregory, R. L., and Wallace, J. (1963), *Recovery From Early Blindness: A Case Study*, Experimental Psychology Society Monograph No. 2, Cambridge: Heffers, 65–129.

Grosrichard, A. (2012), 'An eighteenth-century psychological experiment', in P. Hallward and K. Peden (eds), *Concept and Form, Volume I: Key Texts from the 'Cahiers pour l'analyse'*, London: Verso, 209–27.

Hamilton, R., and Pascual-Leone, A. (1998), 'Cortical plasticity associated with Braille learning', *Trends in Cognitive Science* 2: 168–74.

Hammond, C. (2010), 'SB – The man who was disappointed with what he saw', episode 3 of *Case Study*, transmitted originally on BBC Radio 4 on 25 August 2010, prod. M. Burgess, http://www.bbc.co.uk/programmes/b00tgd1g (accessed 24 September 2015).

Hatfield, G. (1986), 'The senses and the fleshless eye: the Meditations as cognitive exercises', in A. O. Rorty (ed.), *Essays on Descartes' Meditations*, Berkeley: University of California Press, 45–79.

Haüy, V. (1894) [1786], *An Essay on the Education of the Blind*, London: Sampson Low, Marston & Co.

Hebb, D. O. (1949), *The Organization of Behavior: A Neuropsychological Theory*, New York: Wiley.

Heil, J. (1983), *Perception and Cognition*, Berkeley: University of California Press.

Held, R. (2009), 'Visual-haptic mapping and the origin of cross-modal identity', *Optometry and Vision Science* 86(6): 595–8.

Held, R., Ostrovsky, Y., de Gelder, B., Gandhi, T., Ganesh, S., Mathur, U., and Sinha, P. (2011), 'The newly sighted fail to match seen with felt', *Nature Neuroscience* 14: 551–3.

Heller, M. A. (1991), 'Haptic perception in blind people', in M. A. Heller and W. Schiff (eds), *The Psychology of Touch*, London: Lawrence Erlbaum Associates, 239–61.

Heller-Roazen, D. (2007), *The Inner Touch: Archaeology of a Sensation*, Cambridge, MA: MIT Press.

Hollins, M. (1989), *Understanding Blindness: An Integrated Approach*, Hillsdale, NJ: Lawrence Erlbaum Publishers.

Holman, J. (1822), *A Narrative of a Journey Undertaken in the Years 1819, 1820, 1821*, London: F. C. and J. Rivington.

Holman, J. (1834), *Voyage Around the World, including Travels in Africa, Asia, Australasia, America*, Vol. I, London: Smith, Elder & Co.

Holman, J. (1840), *Travels in China, New Zealand, New South Wales, Van Diemen's Land, Cape Horn*, 2nd edition, London: George Routledge.

Hopkins, R. (2005), 'Thomas Reid on Molyneux's question', *Pacific Philosophical Quarterly* 86: 340–64.

Hubbard, P. (2002), *Thinking Geographically: Space, Theory, and Contemporary Human Geography*, London: Continuum.

Hull, J. M. (1991), *Touching the Rock: An Experience of Blindness*, London: Arrow Books.

Hull, J. M. (2001), *In the Beginning There Was Darkness*, London: SCM Press.

Hurley, S., and Noë, A. (2003), 'Neuralplasticity and consciousness', *Biological Philosophy* 18: 131–68.

Husson, T.-A. (2001) [1825], 'Reflections on the moral and physical condition of the blind', in *Reflections: The Life and Writing of a Young*

Blind Woman in Post-Revolutionary France, ed. Catherine J. Kudlick and Zina Weygand, New York: New York University Press, 15–66.

Israel, J. I. (2002), *Radical Enlightenment: Philosophy and the Making of Modernity 1650–1750*, Oxford: Oxford University Press.

Jacomuzzi, A. C., Kobau, P., and Bruno, N. (2003), 'Molyneux's question redux', *Phenomenology and the Cognitive Sciences* 2: 255–80.

James, T. W., James, G. K. H., et al. (2006), 'Do visual and tactile object representations share the same neural substrate?', in M. A. Heller and S. Ballesteros (eds), *Touch and Blindness: Psychology and Neuroscience*, Mahwah, NJ: Lawrence Erlbaum Associates.

James, W. (1927) [1890], *The Principles of Psychology*, New York: Henry Holt & Co.

Jampel, R. S. (1988), 'The four eras in the evolution of cataract surgery', in R. L. Kwitko and C. D. Kelman (eds), *The History of Modern Cataract Surgery*, The Hague: Kugler Publications, 17–33.

Jay, M. (1988), 'Scopic regimes of modernity', in H. Foster (ed.), *Vision and Visuality*, New York: The New Press, 3–27.

Jay, M. (1994), *Downcast Eyes: The Denigration of Vision in Twentieth-Century French Thought*, Berkeley: University of California Press.

Jonas, H. (1954), 'The nobility of sight', *Philosophy and Phenomenological Research* 14(4): 507–19.

Jones, B. (1975), 'Spatial perception in the blind', *British Journal of Psychology* 66(4): 461–72.

Josipovici, G. (1996), *Touch: An Essay*, New Haven, CT: Yale University Press.

Judovitz, D. (1993), 'Vision, representation, and technology in Descartes', in D. M. Levin (ed.), *Modernity and the Hegemony of Vision*, Berkeley: University of California Press, 63–86.

Jütte, R. (2005), *A History of the Senses: From Antiquity to Cyberspace*, trans. J. Lynn, Cambridge: Polity.

Karlsson, G., and Magnusson, A.-K. (1994), 'A phenomenological–psychological investigation of blind people's orientation and mobility', Report 783 from Department of Psychology, Stockholm University, 1–22.

Kauffman, T., Theoret, H., et al. (2002), 'Braille character discrimination in blindfolded human subjects', *NeuroReport* 13: 1–4.

Keeley, B. L. (2002), 'Making sense of the senses: individuating modalities in humans and other animals', *Journal of Philosophy* 99(1): 5–28.

Keeley, B. L. (2009), 'The role of neurobiology in differentiating the senses', in *Oxford Handbook of Philosophy and Neuroscience*, ed. J. Bickle, Oxford: Oxford University Press.

Keller, H. (2003) [1908], *The World I Live In*, ed. R. Shattuck, New York: NYRB Classics.

Keller, H. (2005) [1903], *The Story of My Life*, New York: Pocket Books

Kemp, S., and Fletcher, G. J. O. (1993), 'The medieval theory of the inner senses', *American Journal of Psychology* 106(4): 559–76.

Kennedy, J. M., Gabias, P., and Heller, M. A. (1992), 'Space, haptics and the blind', *Geoforum* 23(2): 175–89.
Kirchner, H., and S. J. Thorpe (2006), 'Ultra-rapid object detection with saccadic eye movements: visual processing speed revisited', *Vision Research* 46: 1762–76.
Kitchin, R. M., Blades, M., and Golledge, R. G. (1997), 'Understanding spatial concepts at the geographic scale without the use of vision', *Progress in Human Geography* 21(2): 225–42.
Klatzky, R. L. (1998), 'Allocentric and egocentric spatial representations: definitions, distinctions, and interconnections', in *Proceedings, Spatial Cognition, An Interdisciplinary Approach to Representing and Processing Spatial Knowledge*, Berlin: Springer, 1–18.
Klatzky, R., and Lederman, S. J. (2003), 'The haptic identification of everyday life objects', in Y. Hatwell, A. Streri, and E. Gentaz (eds), *Touching for Knowing*, Amsterdam: John Benjamins, 105–22.
Klatzky, R. L., Lederman, S. J., et al. (1985), 'Identifying objects by touch: an "expert system"', *Perception & Psychophysics* 37: 299–302.
Kleege, G. (1999), *Sight Unseen*, New Haven, CT: Yale University Press.
Kleege, G. (2005), 'Blindness and visual culture: an eyewitness account', *Journal of Visual Culture* 4(2): 179-90.
Knight, D. (2006), 'In fictional shoes: mental simulation and fiction', in N. Carrol and J. Choi (eds), *Philosophy of Film and Motion Pictures: An Anthology*, Oxford: Blackwell, 271–80.
Koestler, F. (1976), *The Unseen Minority: A Social History of Blindness in America*, New York: David Mckay.
Kupers, R., Pappens, M., et al. (2007), 'rTMS of the occipital cortex abolishes Braille reading and repetition priming in blind subjects', *Neurology* 68: 691–3.
Kurson, R. (2007), *Crashing Through: A True Story of Risk, Adventure, and the Man Who Dared to See*, New York: Random House.
Lebars, J. (1913), 'Epée, Charles-Michel de l'', in *The Catholic Encyclopedia : An International Work of Reference on the Constitution, Doctrine, Discipline, and History of the Catholic Church*, ed. C. G. Herbermann et al., Vol. V, New York: The Encyclopedia Press.
Lederman, S. J., Klatzky, R. L., Chataway, C., and Summers, C. D. (1990), 'Visual mediation and the haptic recognition of two-dimensional pictures of common objects', *Perception & Psychophysics* 47: 54–64.
Leibniz, G. W. F. (1996) [1765], *New Essays on Human Understanding*, ed. P. Remnant and J. Bennett, Cambridge: Cambridge University Press.
Lenay, C., Gapenne, O., et al. (2003), 'Sensory substitution: limits and perspectives', in Y. Hatwell, A. Streri, and E. Gentaz (eds), *Touching for Knowing: Cognitive Psychology of Haptic Manual Perception*, Amsterdam/Philadelphia: John Benjamins.
Lévy-Bruhl, L. (1899), 'The Encyclopaedists', *The Open Court: A Monthly Magazine* 13(3): 129–49.

Lindberg, D. (1976), *Theories of Vision from Al-Kindi to Kepler*, Chicago: University of Chicago Press.

Locke, J. (1991) [1690], *An Essay Concerning Human Understanding* [abridged], London: Everyman.

Loomis, J. M. (1981), 'On the tangibility of letters and Braille', *Perception and Psychophysics* 29: 37–46.

Lotze, R. H. (1885), *Microcosmus: An Essay Concerning Man and His Relation to the World*, 2 vols., trans. E. Hamilton and E. E. Constance Jones, Edinburgh: T. & T. Clark.

Lyon, J. (1976), 'The "Initial Discourse" to Buffon's "Histoire naturelle": the first complete English translation', *Journal of the History of Biology* 9(1): 133–81.

Mackie, J. L. (1976), *Problems from Locke*, Oxford: Oxford University Press.

Magee, B., and Milligan, M. (1998), *Sight Unseen: Letters Between Bryan Magee and Martin Milligan*, London: Phoenix.

Marks, L. E. (1978), *The Unity of the Senses: Interrelations Among the Modalities*, London: Academic Press.

Martin, M. G. F. (1992), 'Sight and touch', in T. Crane (ed.), *The Contents of Experience*, Cambridge: Cambridge University Press.

McDonough, J. K. (2016), 'Descartes' "Dioptrics" and "Optics"', in *The Cambridge Descartes Lexicon*, ed. Larry Nolan, Cambridge: Cambridge University Press, n.p. (in press).

McWilliam, C. (2010), *What To Look For in Winter: A Memoir in Blindness*, New York: HarperCollins.

Mellor, C. M. (2006), *Louis Braille: A Touch of Genius*, Boston: National Braille Press.

Meltzoff, A. N., and Borton, R. W. (1979), 'Intermodal matching by human neonates', *Nature* 282: 403–4.

Merabet, L., and Pascual-Leone, A. (2010), 'Neural reorganization following sensory loss: the opportunity of change', *Nature Reviews Neuroscience* 11: 44–52.

Mérian, J.-B. (2012) [1772], 'The history of Molyneux's problem', in P. Hallward and K. Peden (eds), *Concept and Form, Volume I: Key Texts from the 'Cahiers pour l'analyse'*, London: Verso, 220–7.

Merleau-Ponty, M. (1992) [1945], *The Phenomenology of Perception*, trans. C. Smith, London: Routledge.

Merry, R. V. (1937), 'Fingers for eyes: the story of raised print', *The Scientific Monthly* 44(3): 273–9.

Michalko, R. (1998), *The Mystery of the Eye and the Shadow of Blindness*, London: University of Toronto Press.

Michalko, R. (2002), *The Difference That Disability Makes*, Philadelphia: Temple University Press.

Millar, S. (2006), 'Processing spatial information from touch and movement: implications from and for neuroscience', in M. A. Heller and S.

Ballesteros (eds), *Touch and Blindness: Psychology and Neuroscience*, Mahwah, NJ: Lawrence Erlbaum Associates, 25–48.
Milton, J. (1866), *The Poetical Works of John Milton*, Vol. III, London: Bell and Daldy.
Mitchell, W. J. T. (2002), 'Showing seeing: a critique of visual culture', *Journal of Visual Culture* 1(2): 165–81.
Moisse, K. (2011), 'Like a bat, blind man uses sound to "see"', ABC News website, 26 May 2011, http: //abcnews.go.com/Health/MindMoodNews/blind-man-echolocation/story?id=13684073 (accessed 1 August 2012).
Molyneux, W. (1688), Letter to John Locke, 7 July, in *The Correspondence of John Locke*, ed. E. S. de Beer, Oxford: Clarendon Press, 1978, Vol. III, no. 1064.
Morgan, M. J. (1977), *Molyneux's Question: Vision, Touch and the Philosophy of Perception*, Cambridge: Cambridge University Press
Morley, J. (1878), *Diderot and the Encyclopaedists*, New York: Scribner & Welford.
National Institute of Health (2008), 'Leading causes of blindness', *MedicinePlus Magazine* 3(3): 14–15
Newton, I. (1730) [1704], *Opticks: Or, A Treatise of the Reflections, Refractions, Inflections and Colours of Light*, 4th edition, London: William Innys.
Noë, A. (2004), *Action in Perception*, Cambridge, MA: MIT Press.
Noë, A. (2009), *Out of Our Heads: Why You Are Not Your Brain, and Other Lessons from the Biology of Consciousness*, New York: Hill & Wang.
O'Neill, J. C. (1996), *The Authority of Experience: Sensationist Theory in the French Enlightenment*, State College, PA: Pennsylvania State University Press.
Oliphant, J. (2008), ' "Touching the light": the invention of literacy for the blind', *Paedagogica Historica* 44(1–2): 67–82.
O'Shaughnessy, B. (1989), 'The sense of touch', *Australasian Journal of Philosophy* 67(1): 37–58.
Ostrovsky, Y. A., Andalman, A., and Sinha, P. (2006), 'Vision following extended congenital blindness', *Psychological Science* 17(12): 1009–14.
Pascual-Leone, A., and Hamilton, R. (2001), 'The metamodal organization of the brain', *Progress in Brain Research* 134: 427–45.
Pascual-Leone, A., Amedi, A., et al. (2005), 'The plastic human brain cortex', *Annual Review of Neuroscience* 28: 377–401.
Pascual-Leone, A., Theoret, H., et al. (2006), 'The role of visual cortex in tactile processing: a metamodal brain', in M. A. Heller and S. Ballesteros (eds), *Touch and Blindness: Psychology and Neuroscience*, Mahwah, NJ: Lawrence Erlbaum Associates, 171–96.
Paterson, M. (2006a), ' "Seeing with the hands": blindness, touch and the Enlightenment spatial imaginary', *British Journal of Visual Impairment* 24(2): 52–60.

Paterson, M. (2006b), 'Seeing with the hands, touching with the eyes: vision, touch and the Enlightenment spatial imaginary', *The Senses and Society* 1(2): 224–42.
Paterson, M. (2007), *The Senses of Touch: Haptics, Affects and Technologies*, London: Bloomsbury Academic.
Paterson, M. (2013), 'On "inner touch" and the moving body: *aisthêsis*, kinaesthesis, and aesthetics', in S. Zubarik and G. Ekert (eds), *Touching and to be Touched: Kinesthesia and Empathy in Dance*, Berlin: Walter de Gruyter, 113–29.
Paulson, W. R. (1987), *The Enlightenment, Romanticism and the Blind in France*, Princeton: Princeton University Press.
Piaget, J., and Inhelder, B. (1956), *The Child's Conception of Space*, London: Routledge & Kegan Paul.
Piaget, J., and Inhelder, B. (1969), *The Psychology of the Child*, New York: Basic Books.
Piaget, J., and Inhelder, B. (1971), *Mental Imagery in the Child: A Study of the Development of Imaginal Representation*, New York: Basic Books.
Piveteau, J. (1995), 'Georges-Louis Leclerc, count de Buffon', *Encyclopaedia Britannica*, http: //www.britannica.com/EBchecked/topic/83673/Georges-Louis-Leclerc-count-de-Buffon (accessed 28 October 2012).
Plato (1977), *The Symposium*, trans. W. Hamilton, Harmondsworth: Penguin.
Porter, R. (2003), *Blood and Guts: A Short History of Medicine*, Harmondsworth: Penguin.
Potok. A. (2007) [1980], *Ordinary Daylight: Portrait of an Artist Going Blind*, New York: Bantam Dell.
Ptito, M., Moesgaard, S. M., et al. (2005), 'Cross-modal plasticity revealed by electrotactile stimulation of the tongue in the congenitally blind', *Brain* 128: 606–14.
Quinodoz, D. (2003), *Words That Touch: A Psychoanalyst Learns to Speak*, London: Karnac Books.
Ramachandran, V. S., and Blakeslee, S. (1998), *Phantoms in the Brain: Probing the Mysteries of the Human Mind*, London: HarperCollins.
Rauschecker, J., and Kniepert, U. (1994), 'Auditory localization behaviour in visually deprived cats', *European Journal of Neuroscience* 6: 149–60.
Reid, T. (2000) [1764], *An Inquiry Into the Human Mind on the Principles of Common Sense*, ed. D. R. Brookes, Edinburgh: Edinburgh University Press.
Renier, L., Collignon, O., Poirier, C., Tranduy, D., Vanlierde, A., Bol, A., Veraart, C., and De Volder, A. G. (2005), 'Cross-modal activation of visual cortex during depth perception using auditory substitution of vision', *Neuroimage* 26(2): 573–80.
Révész, G. (1937), 'The problem of space with particular emphasis on specific sensory spaces', *American Journal of Psychology* 50: 429–44.
Révész, G. (1950), *Psychology and Art of the Blind*, London: Longmans.

Riskin, J. (2002), *Science in the Age of Sensibility: The Sentimental Empiricists of the French Enlightenment*, Chicago: University of Chicago Press.

Roberts, J. (2006), *A Sense of the World: How a Blind Man Became History's Greatest Traveller*, London: Simon & Schuster.

Rodas, J. M. (2009), 'On blindness', *Journal of Literary & Cultural Disability Studies* 3(2): 115–30.

Röder, B., and Rösler, F. (2004), 'Compensatory plasticity as a consequence of sensory loss', in G. Clavert, C. Spence, and B. Stein (eds), *The Handbook of Multisensory Processes*, Cambridge, MA: MIT Press, 719–48.

Rolls, G. (2010), *Classic Case Studies in Psychology*, 2nd edition, London: Routledge.

Rorty, R. (1979), *Philosophy and the Mirror of Nature*, Princeton: Princeton University Press.

Rousseau, J.-J. (1979) [1762], *Emile: On Education*, trans. Allan Bloom, New York: Basic Books.

Rubin, B. M. (2009), 'Out of touch with Braille', *Chicago Tribune*, 13 April, Section 1, 8.

Sacks, O. W. (1995), 'To see and not to see', in *An Anthropologist on Mars: Seven Paradoxical Tales*, London: Picador, 102–44.

Sacks, O. W. (2003), 'A neurologist's notebook: the mind's eye – what the blind see', *New Yorker*, 28 July, 48–59.

Sacks, O. W. (2010), *The Mind's Eye*, London: Picador.

Sampaio, E. (1995), 'Les substitutions sensorielles adaptées aux déficits visuels importants', in A. B. Safran and A. Assmacopoulos (eds), *Le déficit visuel. Des fondements neurophysiologiques à la réadaptation*, Paris, Masson, 197–211.

Sampaio, E., Maris, S., et al. (2001), 'Brain plasticity: "visual" acuity of blind persons via the tongue', *Brain Research* 908(2): 204–7.

Saunderson, N. (1741), *The Elements of Algebra, in Ten Books*, ed. J. Saunderson, Vol. I, Cambridge: Cambridge University Press.

Schor, N. (1999), 'Blindness as metaphor', *Differences: A Journal of Feminist Cultural Studies* 11(2): 76–105.

Seigel, J. P. (1995), 'The Enlightenment and the evolution of a language of signs in France and England', in N. S. Struever (ed.), *Language and the History of Thought*, Rochester, NY: University of Rochester Press, 91–110.

Smith, C. (2010), 'BrainPort device lets blind soldier "see" with his tongue', *Huffington Post* 19 May, http: //www.huffingtonpost.com/2010/03/19/brain-port-craig-lundberg_n_505818.html (accessed 1 August 2012).

Smith, M. (1995), *Engaging Characters: Fiction, Emotion and the Cinema*, Oxford: Oxford University Press.

Smith, R. (1738), *A Compleat System of Opticks in Four Books, viz. A Popular, a Mathematical, a Mechanical and a Philosophical Treatise*, Cambridge: Cornelius Crownfield.

Smith, R. (1997), *The Norton History of the Human Sciences*, New York: W.W. Norton.

Sophocles (1984), *The Three Theban Plays: Antigone, Oedipus the King, Oedipus at Colonus*, trans. R. Fagles, Harmondsworth: Penguin.
Spelke, E. S. (1998), 'Nativism, empiricism, and the origins of knowledge', *Infant Behavior and Development* 21: 181–200.
Spence, C., and Driver, J. (2004), *Crossmodal Space and Crossmodal Attention*, Oxford: Oxford University Press.
staff writer (2009), 'Electronic lollipop "allowing blind people to see with their tongues"', *Daily Telegraph*, 1 September, http: //www.telegraph.co.uk/news/newstopics/howaboutthat/6124858/Electronic-lollipop-allowing-blind-people-to-see-with-their-tongues.html (accessed 14 July 2014).
Standage, T. (2002), *The Mechanical Turk: The True Story of the Chess-Playing Machine That Fooled the World*, London: Allen Lane.
Steele, R. (1898), 'White's chocolate-house, August 15th', *The Tatler* 55 (13–16 August 1709), reprinted in *The Tatler*, ed. G. A. Aitken, London: Duckworth, Vol. II, 41–6.
Stewart, S. A. (2002), *Poetry and the Fate of the Senses*, Chicago: University of Chicago Press.
Streri, A., and Gentaz, E. (2004), 'Cross-modal recognition of shape from hand to eyes and handedness in human newborns', *Neuropsychologia* 42(10): 1365–9.
Summerton, N. (2008), *Medicine and Healthcare in Roman Britain*, Princes Risborough: Osprey Publishing.
Suttorp-Schulten, M. S., and Rothova, A. (1996), 'The possible impact of uveitis in blindness: a literature survey', *British Journal of Ophthalmology* 80: 844–8.
Thaler, L., Arnott, S. R., et al. (2011), 'Neural correlates of natural human echolocation in early and late blind echolocation experts', *PLoS ONE*, e20162 DOI: 10.1371/journal.pone.0020162
Titchener, E. B. (1908), *Lectures on the Elementary Psychology of Feeling and Attention*, New York: Macmillan.
Titchener, E. B. (ed.) (1916), *A Beginner's Psychology*. New York: Macmillan.
Tunstall, K. E. (2011), *Blindness and Enlightenment: An Essay*, London: Continuum.
Valvo, A. (1971), *Sight Restoration after Long-term Blindness: The Problems and Behavior Patterns of Visual Rehabilitation*, New York: American Foundation for the Blind.
Van Brussel, L., Gerits, A., et al. (2011), 'Evidence for cross-modal plasticity in adult mouse visual cortex following monocular enucleation', *Cerebral Cortex* 21: 2133–46.
Villey, P. (1930), *The World of The Blind: A Psychological Study*, trans. A. Hallard, London: Duckworth.
Visell, Y. (2009), 'Tactile sensory substitution: models for enaction in HCI', *Interacting with Computers* 21(1–2): 38–53.

Voltaire (1884) [1764], 'Imagination', *A Philosophical Dictionary*, London: W. Dugdale, Vol. II, 45–51.
Voltaire (1904) [1764], 'Distance', in *The Works of Voltaire: A Contemporary Version*, ed. T. Smollett, trans. W. F. Fleming. Akron, OH: The Werner Company, Vol. VIII, 134–44.
Voltaire (1991) [1738], *The Elements of Sir Isaac Newton's Philosophy*, trans. J. A. Hanna, Birmingham: Classics of Opthalmology Library.
Voltaire (1992), 'Elements de philosophie de Newton', in *Oeuvres completes*, Oxford: Alden Press, Vol. XV, 183–652.
Von Senden, M. (1960) [1932], *Space and Sight: The Perception of Space and Shape in the Congenitally Blind before and after Operation*, trans. P. Heath, London: Methuen.
Wade, N. J., and Gregory, R. L. (2006a), 'Editorial essay: Molyneux's answer I', *Perception* 35: 1437–40.
Wade, N. J., and Gregory, R. L. (2006b), 'Editorial essay: Molyneux's answer II', *Perception* 35: 1579–82.
Wait, W. B. (1868), 'Report of the superintendent', *Annual Report of the Board of Managers*, New York Institute for the Education of the Blind, New York: George F. Nesbitt, Vol. XXXII, 7–42.
Weygand, Z. (2009), *The Blind in French Society from the Middle Ages to the Century of Louis Braille*, trans. E.-J. Cohen, Stanford: Stanford University Press.
Wicab.com (2011), 'Select news and media', http://www.wicab.com/en_us/press.html (accessed 12 October 2015).
Wilson, A. M. (1972), *Diderot*, Oxford: Oxford University Press.
Wilson, F. R. (1999), *The Hand: How Its Use Shapes the Brain, Language, and Human Culture*, New York: Vintage.
Winn, M. (1959), 'Mr. Bradford's brave new world', *Daily Express*, 7 January, 7.
Wispé, L. (1990), 'History of the concept of empathy', in N. Eisenberg and J. Strayer (eds), *Empathy and its Development*, Cambridge: Cambridge University Press, 17–37.
World Health Organization (2010), 'Global data on visual impairment', http://www.who.int/blindness/publications/globaldata/en/index.html (accessed 8 June 2013).
World Health Organization (2012), 'Visual impairment and blindness', Factsheet Number 282, http://www.who.int/mediacentre/factsheets/fs282/en/index.html (accessed 8 June 2013).
Yolton, J. (1984), *Perceptual Acquaintance from Descartes to Reid*, Minneapolis: University of Minnesota Press.

Index

l'Abbé de l'Epée, 139, 141, 145, 146
abstraction (propensity for), 12, 51, 73, 136, 169, 173, 174, 177, 178
active touch, 106, 166, 167; *see also* Gibson, James J.
Addition á la lettre sur les aveugles (Diderot), 87, 99, 108, 122, 132–6, 140
age-related macular degeneration (AMD), 13; *see also* macular degeneration
d'Alembert, Jean le Rond, 102–3, 113, 129, 136, 153
American Foundation for the Blind (AFB), 12
Aristotle, 21, 36, 37, 54, 120, 202
arithmetic, 116, 135, 143, 145, 148, 152
aveuglement, 136; *see also cecité*
aveugle-né, 7, 10, 11, 104, 117, 129, 131, 136
aveugles-operé, 7

Bach-y-Rita, Paul, 19, 29, 44, 111, 162, 167–78
Barbier, Charles, 154–6
Berkeley, George, 16, 17, 32–5, 41, 44–9, 51–4, 71–6, 80, 82, 85, 88–94, 96, 99, 106, 109, 112, 131, 141, 163, 166
Essay Towards a New Theory of Vision, 16, 32, 44, 46–9, 71, 163
blindness
and abstraction, 12, 51, 73, 136, 169, 173, 174, 177, 178
as *aveuglement*, 136
as blank figure, 9–11, 99, 104, 189, 205
as *cecité*, 135–6, 143–4
as darkness, 5, 14–17, 37, 39, 59–60, 114, 116, 127, 135–6, 140–1, 142, 144, 153, 184–7, 189–93, 195, 197–201, 205–6
as hypothetical, 9–11

as lack, 4, 15, 126, 135, 141, 192, 194, 206–8
as night, 24, 39, 73, 107, 141–2, 184, 186, 190, 195, 199–200
question of, 1–21
and testimony, 11, 18, 109–22, 188
and vision impairment, 12–15
as visual deprivation, 15, 144, 174–81
Blind Traveller, 184–5, 199–204, 206; *see also* Holman, James
Borges, Jorge Luis, 20, 184, 186, 188–9, 195–7, 199–201
Boston Line Letter, 151
Bradford, Sidney, 57–67, 74, 83, 206; *see also* S.B.
Braille (writing and reading system), 18–19, 31–2, 55, 111, 122, 134, 137–9, 150–3, 155–60
Braille, Louis, 155–7
BrainPort™, 111, 160–2, 165, 170–1, 182
Buffon, George-Louis Leclerc, Comte de, 16–18, 46, 69, 82, 85, 87–9, 93, 95, 97, 99, 101–8, 117
  Premier discours, 102–3, 106, 117

Cabanis, Pierre Jean George, 86
Café des Aveugles, 145–7, 149
camera obscura, 16, 37–8, 44

cane (visual aid), 1, 19, 26–8, 31–2, 60, 66, 80, 136, 162, 175, 177
Cassirer, Ernst, 16–17, 33, 46, 85–8, 90–2, 109
cataract (removal), 2, 7, 10, 13, 33, 39–49, 55, 58, 67–76, 86–90, 95, 103–9, 119, 132, 136, 199
  unbandaging, 61, 63, 73, 117, 129, 132
  see also couching
cecité, 135–6, 143–4; *see also aveuglement*
Charles Bonnet Syndrome, 192, 203
Châtelet, Madame du, 112
Cheselden, William, 7–8, 10–11, 17–18, 34, 41–2, 49, 52, 58–9, 61, 64–9, 72–6, 78–9, 82–3, 85–8, 90, 92–6, 101, 103, 105–8, 110–11, 114–18, 129, 131, 139–40, 189
Cicero, 184, 196–9
common sensibles, 45, 54
Condillac, 8, 17, 33, 69, 72, 82, 85–6, 90–1, 96, 98–101, 103–5, 109, 115, 117–18, 120, 129, 131, 136, 138, 140, 143
  Essai sur l'origine des connaisances humaines, 8, 85, 99–100, 131
  Traité des Sensations, 85–6, 90, 98–102, 117, 120, 129, 131

Consolatio, 194, 197
couching, 39, 68, 86–7, 106, 117;
   see also cataract (removal)

Daviel, Jacques, 7, 82, 86–7,
   95, 132
De rerum natura (Lucretius),
   102, 128
Democritus, 196
Derrida, Jacques, 190, 199–200,
   206
Descartes, René, 1, 3, 7, 16–37,
   40, 46, 54–8, 67, 85–6,
   89–93, 97, 105, 108–9, 116,
   119–20, 160, 170, 199
   Dioptrique, 1, 3, 16, 21–6,
     29–34, 37, 40, 46, 58, 86,
     93, 170, 189
   Meditations on First
     Philosophy, 25, 91–3
diabetes, 14, 202
Dictionnaire Philosophique
   (Voltaire), 46, 88, 95
Diderot, Denis, 1–3, 9, 11, 16–18,
   29–34, 51, 56, 66, 69, 81,
   85–91, 95–104, 108–45,
   152–3, 189, 195, 198
   and *Addition á la lettre sur les*
     aveugles (Diderot), 87, 99,
     108, 122, 132–6, 140
   and blind man of Puiseaux, 18,
     29–30, 66, 100, 111, 113–25,
     128, 132, 136, 140, 189
   and the *Encyclopédie*, 1, 94,
     102, 129, 136, 153
   and *Lettre sur les aveugles*,
     2, 9, 11, 18, 29–31, 51,
     85–9, 97–8, 108–45,
     189, 198
Dioptrique (Descartes), 1, 3, 16,
   21–6, 29–34, 37, 40, 46, 58,
   86, 93, 170, 189

echolocation, 175, 217; *see also*
   Kish, Daniel
Electronic Travel Aids, 11, 162,
   182, 192
Éléments de la philosophie de
   Newton (Voltaire), 8, 17, 69,
   85, 87–90, 95–103
Elements of Algebra
   (Saunderson), 124, 126–7
embossed script, 18, 138, 143,
   149–51, 153, 156–9
Émile, 142
empathy, 15, 19, 184–8, 194,
   205
Encyclopédie (Diderot and
   d'Alembert), 1, 94, 102, 129,
   136, 153
episteme, 15–18
Essai sur l'education des aveugles
   (Haüy), 19, 146–9, 155
Essai sur l'origine des
   connaisances humaines
   (Condillac), 8, 85, 99–100,
   131
Essay Concerning Human
   Understanding, An (Locke),
   6–7, 34, 36–44, 74, 86

Essay Towards a New Theory of Vision, An (Berkeley), 16, 34, 46–9, 71, 163

facial recognition, 62
facial vision, 204
fingertips, 14, 30–1, 116, 134, 142–3, 150, 158–60, 171, 198
Foucault, Michel, 5–8, 59, 109, 117–18, 141
fovea, 14, 31, 120, 158–9
Freud, Sigmund, 6, 186–7, 196
Friel, Brian, 84

Gallagher, Shaun, 33, 54, 56
Garland-Thomson, Rosemarie, 4, 11, 185–7, 205
Getaz, Joan, 80
Gibson, James J., 80, 166–7, 172–4, 178
glaucoma, 13, 86
Grant, Roger (Oculist), 17, 71–2, 86, 110
Gregory, Richard D., 17, 29, 40–4, 57–68, 78–9, 82–4, 91, 187
Grosrichard, Alain, 7–8, 11–12, 34

habitual custom (Locke), 36, 40, 44, 53
haptic, 19, 26, 63–5, 105, 111, 121, 125, 158, 164, 166, 179–81, 185, 188, 199, 203–6

haptocentric, 192–3, 203–6; *see also* ocularcentric
Haüy, Valentin, 18–19, 138–54
 Essai sur l'education des aveugles, 19, 146–9, 155
Helmholtz, Hermann von, 97
Holman, James, 184–5, 201–6; *see also* Blind Traveller
Hooke, Robert, 37, 99
Howe, Samuel Gridley, 154
H.S. (case study), 59, 81–2
Hull, John, 15, 20, 187–9, 191–5, 199–200, 203–6
Husson, Thérèse-Adèle, 12
hypothetical blind man, 3, 9–10, 16, 20, 26–9, 33, 41, 98, 109, 114, 124, 129, 189, 195, 197, 202; *see also* Kleege, Georgina

in relievo, 148, 150, 155; *see also* embossed script
inner vision, 187, 202
Institut Royale des Jeunes Aveugles, 153–7

James, William, 64, 78–9

Keller, Helen, 12, 19–20, 110, 184, 189, 191, 197–200, 203–6
Kempelen, Wolfgang von, 148, 150
kinaesthesia, 80–1, 163, 192
King Lear, 204

Kish, Daniel, 175; *see also* echolocation
Kleege, Georgina, 9–10, 14–15, 20, 189–91, 197, 200–1, 205, 215; *see also* hypothetical blind man

La Mettrie, Julian Offray de, 8, 17, 33, 85, 99, 112, 118, 126
Le Sueur, Francois, 148–9
Leibniz, Gottfried Wilhelm, 33, 37, 45, 50–3, 77–8, 119, 140
Lettre sur les aveugles (Diderot), 2, 9, 11, 18, 29–31, 51, 85–9, 97–8, 108–45, 189, 198
Locke, John, 3, 6, 10–11, 16–17, 32–55, 64, 67, 71–5, 82, 85–101, 109, 119–20, 128, 138–9, 143, 161, 163, 189
  Essay Concerning Human Understanding, 6–7, 34, 36–44, 74, 86
lollipop, 170–4, 178, 182; *see also* TDU

macular degeneration, 13, 20, 189, 201–2; *see also* age-related macular degeneration
May, Michael, 59, 62, 66; *see also* M.M.
Meditations on First Philosophy (Descartes), 25, 91–3
Mérian, Johann Bernhard, 140–2, 144
Michalko, Rod, 259, 262, 270, 306

Milton, John, 255, 263, 278, 279, 287, 306
  and *Samson Agonistes*, 190, 200
M.M. (case study), 59; *see also* May, Michael
Molyneux, William, 6, 34, 40, 189
Molyneux problem, 3, 6–11, 16–19, 28–9, 32–58, 63–4, 71–81, 85–6, 89–90, 93, 96, 99–100, 109–11, 115–18, 128–9, 134, 136–40, 142–3, 160–4, 167, 172, 183, 189

Nancy, Jean-Luc, 199
neonate (blind), 18, 54, 64–5, 98, 104–6, 176; *see also* newborn infant
neuroplasticity, 175–9, 182–3
New York Point, 156
newborn infant (blind), 104, 129–31; *see also* neonate
Newton, Isaac, 8, 38, 40, 87–9, 104, 112, 119, 128
NLP (No Light Perception), 2, 4, 12, 14
noctograph, 154–5, 202–3
normate (body), 11, 205–6

ocular surgery, 8, 11, 18, 72, 83, 118; *see also* cataract surgery; couching
ocularcentric, 21
oculomotor, 62–3, 77, 177
optic flow, 172, 176

optic nerve, 12–13, 23, 27, 32, 176, 202

Paradis, Teresia von, 60, 82, 134, 136, 144–5, 148–53
Perkins Institute, 110, 151, 156
Philosophes, 44, 101, 117, 139
Pignier, Alexandre René, 154–5
plasticity, 58, 79, 162–4, 171, 175–83; *see also* neuroplasticity
Plato, 21, 196, 202
prehensile hand, 198–200
Premier discours (Buffon), 102–3, 106, 117
Puiseaux, blind man of, 18, 29–30, 66, 100, 111, 113–25, 128, 132, 136, 140, 189; *see also* Diderot

Reid, Thomas, 16, 33–5, 50–5, 163
retinitis pigmentosa (RP), 4, 14, 161
Révész, Géza, 166–7, 178, 181
Rousseau, Jean-Jacques, 98–9, 112, 142, 144, 152
Royal National Institute for the Blind (RNIB), 157

saccades, 62, 77, 177
Sacks, Oliver, 3, 20, 59, 62, 79, 82–4, 185, 189, 192, 204
Samson Agonistes, 190, 200

Saunderson, Nicholas, 18–19, 51–5, 113–18, 123–36, 144, 152–3
and calculating tables, 2, 148, 152–3
Elements of Algebra, 124, 126–7
S.B. (case study), 17, 57–60, 67, 82–3, 185; *see also* Bradford, Sidney
sensationism, 85–6, 98, 101, 109, 115–16, 138
sensory deprivation, 140–1, 175, 182, 206
sensory substitution, 3, 16, 19, 29–32, 44, 55–6, 63, 137, 145, 159–83
Smith-Kettlewell Portable Electrical Stimulation System, 168
Sophocles, 184, 186
spatial perception, 17–18, 44, 49, 69, 76–81, 166, 174, 185, 193
Synge, Edward, 35, 45, 50–1, 53

tactile maps, 153, 160
tactile reading, 143, 158–9
tactile signs, 111, 121, 134–41, 150, 153–5, 160
TDU (Tongue Display Unit), 170–1, 174, 178, 182; *see also* lollipop
testimony (of blind), 11, 18, 109–22, 188

Titchener, Edward Bradford, 64, 188
Torey, Zoltan, 15
Traité des Sensations (Condillac), 85–6, 90, 98–102, 117, 120, 129, 131
TVSS (Tactile Visual Sensory Substitution), 19, 111, 137, 161–83

unbandaging (after cataract removal), 61, 63, 73, 117, 129, 132

Valvo, Alberto, 17, 59, 62, 58, 81–4, 185
Virgil (case study), 59, 62–3, 82–4
vision impairment, 2, 4, 12–15, 20, 135, 189, 192, 205

visual deprivation, 15, 144, 174–81
Voltaire (François-Marie Arouet), 7–8, 16–18, 34, 46, 69, 72, 82–118, 128–9, 133, 136, 138, 143
  Dictionnaire Philosophique (Voltaire), 46, 88, 95
  Éléments de la philosophie de Newton, 8, 17, 69, 85, 87–90, 95–103
von Senden, Marius, 34, 59–61, 68, 79–82, 131–2, 163

WHO (World Health Organization), 4, 12–13
WICAB Corporation, 19, 170

zoom effect, 168, 172